Contemporary Diagnosis and Management of

Pso

John Koo, MD
Director, Psoriasis and Skin Treatment Center
Professor and Vice Chairman
Department of Dermatology
University of California Medical Center
San Francisco, CA

and

Grace D. Bandow, MD
Division of Dermatology
Department of Medicine
Washington University School of Medicine
St. Louis, MO

and

Jane C. Kwan, MD
Dermatologist
Permanente Medical Group
Santa Clara, CA

Second Edition

Published by Medical Learning Systems
Newtown, Pennsylvania, USA

This book has been prepared and is presented as a service to the medical community. The information provided reflects the knowledge, experience, and personal opinions of the authors John Koo, MD, Director, Psoriasis and Skin Treatment Center, and Professor and Vice Chairman, Department of Dermatology, University of California Medical Center, San Francisco, CA; Grace D. Bandow, MD, Division of Dermatology, Department of Medicine, Washington University School of Medicine, St. Louis, MO; and Jane C. Kwan, MD, Dermatologist, Permanente Medical Group, Santa Clara, CA.

This book is not intended to replace or to be used as a substitute for the complete prescribing information prepared by each manufacturer for each drug. Because of possible variations in drug indications, in dosage information, in newly described toxicities, in drug/drug interactions, and in other items of importance, reference to such complete prescribing information is definitely recommended before any of the drugs discussed are used or prescribed.

International Standard Book Number: 978-1-931981-28-6

Library of Congress Catalog Card Number: 2007932791

Second edition

Table of Contents

Chapter 1
Introduction 5

Chapter 2
Diagnosing and Assessing Psoriasis 8

Chapter 3
Types of Psoriasis 12

Chapter 4
Determining Disease Severity 15

Chapter 5
Topical Medications for Psoriasis 18

Chapter 6
Phototherapy 42

Chapter 7
Oral Agents 46

Chapter 8
Inpatient (Goeckerman) Therapy 59

Chapter 9
**Combination, Rotational, and
Sequential Therapies** 62

Chapter 10
**Advances in the Treatment
of Psoriasis: The Biologic Agents** 70

Chapter 11
Nail Psoriasis 84

Chapter 12
Psoriatic Arthritis 86

Chapter 13
Psoriasis in Pregnancy 90

Chapter 14
**For the Nonspecialist:
When to Refer** 94

Index 96

CHAPTER **1**

Introduction

P soriasis is one of the most commonly encountered conditions in dermatology practice and is regularly seen in primary care medicine. In the United States, a recent nationwide survey revealed the prevalence of psoriasis to be between 2.1% and 2.6% of the population. Psoriasis is relatively rare in childhood; patients typically develop the disease in young adulthood. Racially, psoriasis is most prevalent among whites, about half as prevalent in African Americans as compared with whites, and about half as prevalent among Asian Americans as compared with African Americans. Men and women are affected equally.

In most patients, psoriasis is experienced as a pruritic, inflammatory condition with a chronic remitting and relapsing course. In contrast to atopic dermatitis, which tends to improve as the patient ages, psoriasis remains active throughout the patient's lifetime or gradually become more widespread. Also, unlike atopic dermatitis, where the onset of disease is usually limited to childhood or young adulthood, psoriasis can develop at any age. First episodes of psoriasis have even been reported in centenarians.

Although it is known that a predisposition to develop psoriasis can be genetically transmitted, many cases arise in individuals with no reported family history of the disease. Several factors are known to exacerbate psoriasis, including traumatic injury to the skin, physical and psychological stress, cold weather, excessive alcohol intake, and drugs such as lithium and β-blockers. Table 1-1 provides a list of drugs that can exacerbate psoriasis.

Table 1-1: Drugs That Can Exacerbate Psoriasis

- Corticosteroids (rebound can occur upon withdrawal)
- Interferons
- Lithium (Eskalith®, Lithobid®); divalproex (Depakote®); and carbamazepine (Carbatrol®, Epitol®, Tegretol®) are acceptable alternatives to treat bipolar disorder
- β-Blockers
- Nonsteroidal anti-inflammatory drugs (NSAIDs)
- Angiotensin-converting enzyme (ACE) inhibitors
- Antimalarials (chloroquine [Aralen®], hydroxy-chloroquine [Plaquenil®], quinacrine, and others)
- Gemfibrozil (Lopid®)

The pathophysiology of psoriasis involves an abnormal activation of the immune system in the skin. T cells are triggered and release cytokines, which cause inflammation of target tissues and activate more T cells, further propagating an inflammatory cascade. Many of the treatments being used or developed for psoriasis are immunomodulators, which decrease and interfere with lymphocyte activity in psoriatic skin. In addition to inflammation, the epidermis in psoriatic skin reproduces up to 10 times faster than normal, and contains double the normal number of proliferating cells (which produce 30 times more cells per day than healthy skin). This increased rate of cell turnover, coupled with the inflammatory process, results in the typical lesions of psoriasis.

Most patients with psoriasis suffer localized outbreaks (Figure 1-1, see color insert), especially on the elbows, knees, and scalp. However, a small but significant proportion of patients experience generalized psoriasis. Those with localized involvement have the potential to flare, which can then lead to generalized involvement (Figure 1-2, see color insert).

Although skin disorders are often trivialized by those who do not have them, a rigorous study of the impact of psoriasis on health-related quality of life (QOL) using a validated QOL questionnaire revealed that the negative impact of psoriasis is no less than that seen in other serious, chronic medical conditions such as cancer, hypertension, diabetes, arthritis, heart disease, and depression. In fact, only congestive heart failure patients had worse physical QOL scores than psoriasis patients. In terms of impact on mental QOL, only patients with chronic lung disease and major depression scored worse than patients with psoriasis.

Consequently, it is important to learn how to manage psoriasis, not only because of its prevalence, but also because of the profound impact it can have on a patient's QOL. In addition, timely and proper intervention can prevent localized disease from becoming generalized, and, in some rare instances, reduce the risk of conversion into life-threatening erythrodermic or generalized pustular psoriasis. This book describes the diagnosis and management of psoriasis with an emphasis on optimizing treatment by using the full breadth of the therapeutic armamentarium that is now available for psoriasis patients.

Selected Readings

Christophers E, Mroweitz U: Psoriasis. In: Fitzpatrick TB, Freedberg IM, Eisen AZ, et al, eds: *Dermatology in General Medicine*, 5th ed. New York, NY, McGraw-Hill, 1999, pp 495-533.

Rapp SR, Feldman SR, Exum ML, et al: Psoriasis causes as much disability as other major medical illnesses. *J Am Acad Dermatol* 1999;41:401-407.

CHAPTER 2

Diagnosing and Assessing Psoriasis

In most cases, psoriatic lesions can be diagnosed clinically without performing a skin biopsy. They are characterized by the presence of well-demarcated, scaly plaques with sharply defined borders. Psoriatic lesions are typically located on the extensor aspects of the body, such as the elbows and the knees. Other areas of involvement include the scalp (particularly the occipital scalp) behind the ears, umbilicus, lower back, shins, nails, and the gluteal cleft. Gluteal pinking is one of the more characteristic signs of psoriasis. This is the presence of erythema ranging from pink to 'beefy' bright red, within the buttock crease. It often lacks scales because of the moist, occluded nature of the buttock area.

An untreated psoriatic plaque consists of silvery, white, unusually thick, micaceous scales. The term micaceous is derived from the word mica, which is a classification of various minerals that crystallize, thereby allowing perfect cleavage into thin, silvery planes. Micaceous scales are much thicker than those found in other common scaly skin conditions such as seborrheic dermatitis (seborrhea) or atopic dermatitis (eczema). Other chronic inflammatory skin conditions such as seborrheic dermatitis, atopic dermatitis, or other forms of eczema generally lack such sharply demarcated borders. They are instead characterized by lesions with diffuse, poorly defined borders such that the examiner may have difficulty delineating the point between normal and diseased skin.

Nail involvement includes specific findings such as shallow, punctate pits; 'oil spots;' and onycholysis, which help distinguish psoriatic nail involvement from other pathologic nail conditions. These distinguishing characteristics become most important when a patient presents with nail disease only (see Chapter 11). Onycholysis is less specific for psoriasis than nail pitting and oil spots because it is often seen in other traumatic, inflammatory, or ideopathic conditions involving the nail bed.

Although psoriasis is usually an easy diagnosis based on its characteristic features, the differential is important, especially in a primary care setting where most patients present for the first time. Other common diagnoses to be considered include atopic dermatitis, contact dermatitis, seborrheic dermatitis, tinea, candidiasis, pityriasis rosea, drug eruption, cutaneous T-cell lymphoma (mycosis fungoides [MF]), and pityriasis rubra pilaris (PRP).

In contrast to atopic dermatitis, which primary care physicians are likely to see more than any other inflammatory skin disease, psoriasis is distinguishable not only by its morphology, as described above, but also by its location. Unless psoriasis is widespread, it is typically a disease of elbows, knees, gluteal cleft, and scalp. Atopic dermatitis usually involves flexural areas such as antecubital and popliteal fossae. An atopic history, including asthma or allergic rhinitis in either the patient or family members, can also be a clue. Atopic patients often report sensitivity to environmental triggers such as dust, pets, foods, or pollen as well as a susceptibility to secondary bacterial, fungal, and viral infections. Psoriatic skin is usually not particularly sensitive to environmental elements, bacterial overgrowth, or secondary infections. Skin antigen testing will further distinguish psoriatic and atopic skin. Test results tend to demonstrate normal reactivity in psoriatic patients vs an anergic response in atopic patients.

Psoriasis is easily distinguished from seborrheic dermatitis. Seborrheic dermatitis involves only the sebaceous, follicle-rich areas of the scalp, face (the T-zone or eyebrows and the area on and around the nose), ears, central chest, and rarely, central upper back and the groin. Seborrhea is typically poorly demarcated, pink, edematous, oily-appearing skin with yellow-brown scales. On the scalp, the scaling of seborrheic dermatitis tends to be diffuse with fine, greasy scales, commonly called dandruff, while psoriatic scalp involvement demonstrates sharply demarcated plaques typical of the lesions on the body, with much coarser and thicker scaling. On the face, seborrheic dermatitis is typically limited to sebaceous areas around the eyebrows and the nasolabial folds while facial psoriasis is less common altogether, and can be found anywhere on the face. However, clinicians should not assume that a red, scaly rash on the face of a known psoriatic patient is necessarily psoriasis. Facial seborrheic dermatitis does commonly occur in conjunction with psoriasis and is called sebopsoriasis.

Some of the more unusual skin conditions resembling psoriasis include MF, PRP, and a rare form of psoriasis morphologically between psoriasis and eczema called eczematoid psoriasis, or psoriasiform eczema. MF is a slowly progressive form of cutaneous T-cell lymphoma that often mimics and is easily misdiagnosed as either psoriasis or eczema. The diagnosis is made by combining clinical and histologic features and often takes several years before findings become diagnostic. If suspicion is high, or if patients do not respond to treatment, repeat biopsies should be performed because they are frequently nondiagnostic during the early years of the disease. Retrospective studies have shown that a lag time from disease onset to diagnosis ranges from 4 to 10 years. Although MF occurs in any age group, it is often suspected in older patients, especially when the lesions are not as sharply demarcated or micaceous as classic psoriatic lesions.

PRP is a rare skin condition characterized by an explosive onset of highly inflammatory, erythematous, macular lesions originating on the head and descending toward the trunk and eventually the legs. This progression is different from psoriasis in which the face tends to be the last location involved. In fact, the face is spared in most psoriasis patients despite frequent scalp involvement. Patients with PRP usually have an extremely thick, smooth, waxy layer of dead skin cells on their palms and the soles of their feet, giving the appearance that their hands have been dipped in carnauba wax (Figure 2-1, see color insert). This is different from the silvery, flaky hyperkeratosis of psoriasis on the palms and soles. Patients also typically have generalized bright salmon-colored to orange-red erythema on the trunk with characteristic small islands of spared, normal skin. Skin biopsy is helpful in differentiating PRP from psoriasis.

In rare cases, patients present with clinical manifestations consistent with both eczema and psoriasis. The plaques are not as well demarcated as psoriasis, but more demarcated than typical eczema. Scales are also morphologically between the thickness typical of psoriasis and eczema. This diagnosis is rarely made, and patients with features of eczematoid psoriasis or psoriasiform eczema should undergo biopsies to rule out MF.

Another rare clinical manifestation of this mixed state involves hand dermatitis exhibiting both pustules suggestive of pustular psoriasis and 'tapioca' vesicles (ie, small fluid-filled bubbles) of dyshidrotic eczema (Figure 2-2, see color insert). These cases may be preferentially treated with agents that are effective for both psoriasis and eczema, such as topical steroids, ultraviolet B (UVB), or psoralen plus ultraviolet A (PUVA) phototherapy rather than treatment specific to psoriasis, such as calcipotriene (Dovonex®).

Selected Readings

Christophers E, Mroweitz U: Psoriasis. In: Fitzpatrick TB, Freedberg IM, Eisen AZ, et al, eds: *Dermatology in General Medicine*, 5th ed. New York, NY, McGraw-Hill, 1999, pp 495-533.

Epstein EH Jr, Levin DL, Croft JD Jr, et al: Mycosis fungoides. Survival, prognostic features, response to therapy and autopsy findings. *Medicine (Baltimore)* 1972;51:61-72.

CHAPTER 3

Types of Psoriasis

Plaque-type Psoriasis

More than 90% of patients with psoriasis have plaque-type disease. Lesions are sharply demarcated with wide-ranging degrees of erythema, induration, and scaling. When plaque-type psoriasis first erupts, lesions initially appear as tiny, well-demarcated 'islands' of scaly, inflammatory skin, which quickly coalesce to form larger plaques. While plaques can occur on almost any part of the skin (aside from the mucous membranes), they are typically found on the elbows, knees, shins, lower back, umbilicus, and intergluteal fold (Figure 1-1, see color insert). The scalp is commonly involved, especially behind the ears and in the occipital region, while the face is often spared.

Pruritus of varying severity frequently occurs but is not as consistently observed as in patients with atopic dermatitis or other forms of eczema. Some patients with widespread psoriasis experience little itching, while others with localized plaques may suffer from disruptive pruritus. Unlike the itching associated with atopic dermatitis where histamine is thought to play a major role, the pruritus of psoriasis generally does not respond well to nonsedating antihistamines such as loratadine (Alavert®, Claritin®).

Erythrodermic Psoriasis

Erythrodermic psoriasis (Figure 3-1, see color insert) involves most or all of the skin surface, manifesting as a bright erythema that causes the entire body to take on the appearance of a cooked lobster. Any patient with plaque-type psoriasis can quickly convert into erythrodermic psoriasis if he or she experiences a severe flare-up. Unlike plaque-type psoriasis, where systemic symptoms are rare, many erythrodermic psoriasis patients experience uncomfortable symptoms such as fever, chills, and rigors. Erythrodermic psoriasis can be a medical emergency, especially in the elderly. Because of the large area of compromised barrier function, the patient can easily develop a prerenal state. A risk of renal failure or high-output cardiac failure secondary to the substantial shunting of blood to the skin surface is possible. Erythrodermic patients with concomitant medical conditions that are unstable should be treated in an inpatient setting.

Guttate Psoriasis

Guttate psoriasis presents as a sudden, diffuse eruption consisting of smaller, droplet-size lesions on the trunk and extremities (Figure 3-2, see color insert). It tends to occur in young adults and is often preceded by an acute bacterial infection, most commonly streptococcal pharyngitis, or by systemic corticosteroid withdrawal.

Inverse Psoriasis

The patient with inverse psoriasis experiences prominent involvement of the flexural areas, such as the antecubital and popliteal fossae, inframammary region, axillae, inguinal region, groin, and intergluteal fold (Figure 3-3, see color insert). Although these areas are often spared in the typical psoriasis patient, inverse psoriasis can coexist with regular plaque-type psoriasis. The treatment of inverse psoriasis must be carefully conducted because topical agents, such as corticosteroids, can induce atrophy, irritation, and maceration in self-occluded areas of the skin.

Pustular Psoriasis

Pustular psoriasis (Figure 3-4, see color insert) clinically manifests as psoriatic lesions that are filled with sterile pus.

Because of its unique appearance, pustular psoriasis is frequently misdiagnosed as an infectious process. Patients are often kept on antibiotics for a prolonged period before the primary care physician is aware of the actual diagnosis, either through self-discovery or dermatology consultation. Pustular psoriasis is generally more difficult to treat than plaque-type psoriasis and occurs in localized and generalized forms.

Localized pustular psoriasis can be highly disabling, especially when it involves the palms and/or the soles of the feet, but is usually not life-threatening. In contrast, generalized pustular psoriasis, also known as the von Zumbusch type, is a medical emergency and should be treated accordingly. Patients with a generalized pustular flare-up can die of sepsis, renal failure, congestive heart failure, and other complications if the condition is not promptly brought under control. To prevent such sequelae, these patients should be monitored closely and hospitalized as quickly as possible with a dermatologist on consult.

Hand and Foot Psoriasis

Hand and foot psoriasis occurs as either plaque-type or pustular disease that is most severe on the palms and soles (Figures 3-5, 3-6, and 3-7, see color insert). It is challenging to manage, and patients may require systemic therapy in addition to topicals. The thickness of the skin on the palms and soles impairs the ability of topical medications to effectively penetrate down to the living layer of the skin. Although the area affected may be small, the location of the lesions makes hand and foot psoriasis disabling to the patient. As a result, more elaborate and aggressive treatment is often warranted for these patients. Besides the hands and feet, psoriasis affects other areas that require specialized treatment. Cases such as nail psoriasis and scalp psoriasis will be described in further detail in the therapy sections of this handbook.

CHAPTER 4

Determining Disease Severity

P soriasis is classically categorized as mild, moderate, or severe. Usually, mild disease can be controlled with topical agents, while moderate-to-severe cases require the addition of systemic agents. One of the most important decisions that physicians need to make is whether psoriasis can be adequately treated with topical medications alone or whether it requires systemic treatment. This key decision is made with considerations of such factors as the extent of psoriasis in terms of body surface area (BSA) involved, responsiveness or lack of response to topical agents, and the quality-of-life (QOL) impact the disease has on the patient. Another consideration is the presence or absence of psoriatic arthritis.

The palm of one's hand, including the fingers and the thumb (ie, from the wrist to the tip of the fingers), constitutes approximately 1% of the total BSA. If ≥10% of the BSA is involved, it becomes tedious and time consuming to apply topical medications to all areas of involved skin. Although some patients could potentially chase after every psoriatic lesion with topical medications even if a large amount of BSA is involved, most busy, working individuals find it unfeasible to treat >10% of the BSA with topical medications alone. With >10% BSA involvement, it also becomes difficult to obtain a sufficient quantity of topical medications for adequate coverage. Moreover, frequently used topical medications for psoriasis, such as super-potent topical steroids and calcipotriene (Dovonex®), have limitations on the amount of drug that is allowed to be used per unit time for safety reasons. Therefore, any patient with ≥10% BSA involvement should be managed by a dermatologist so that phototherapy and/or systemic therapy can be used in addition to topical treatment.

Even when the BSA involved is <10%, phototherapy or systemic therapy should be considered if the psoriatic lesions prove to be unresponsive to optimized topical therapeutic regimens. This is especially true if the localized involvement is physically disabling or emotionally, occupationally, or socially devastating to the patient. For example, a patient may have a small proportion of BSA affected by psoriasis, but if the hands or feet comprise the involved areas, the impact on QOL may be profound and aggressive intervention warranted. A person whose appearance is important to his or her occupation may find even a single plaque of psoriasis on the face debilitating, even though the disease is not widespread.

Depending on the study cited, a range of 10% to 40% of psoriatic patients have psoriatic arthritis. A major clinical difference between psoriatic arthritis and psoriasis is that even if psoriasis is widespread, the patient is 'as good as new' if it is adequately treated and resolved, because psoriasis generally does not leave permanent scars unless patients excoriate or damage their skin in other ways. However, if the patient is afflicted with psoriatic arthritis severe enough to cause bony changes, the destruction is irreversible, even if the patient is appropriately treated at a later time with antiarthritic agents.

No topical medications are known to help psoriatic arthritis. Therefore, if early signs and symptoms appear, it is best to refer patients to a rheumatologist and prepare them for possible initiation of systemic antipsoriatic medications. In addition to improving the skin, drugs such as etanercept (Enbrel®) can also arrest the destructive progression of psoriatic arthritis and are the agents of choice for those with both skin and joint manifestations.

The Koo-Menter Psoriasis Instrument (KMPI) has been developed to assist physicians in making decisions about whether the psoriasis patient can be adequately treated with topical therapy alone or whether he or she may need phototherapy or a systemic agent in addition to topical therapy. The KMPI is an integrated tool to help physicians perform a comprehensive evaluation of psoriasis patients including physical severity, QOL impact, and arthritis issues, and document the need for a more aggressive treatment.

Ultimately, it is a clinical judgment as to how aggressively the patient needs to be treated, and this decision should be made after taking into account all of the above-mentioned factors.

Selected Readings

Feldman SR, Koo JY, Menter A, et al: Decision points for the initiation of systemic treatment for psoriasis. *J Am Acad Dermatol* 2005;53:101-107.

Koo JY, Kowalski JW, Lebwohl MG, et al: The Koo-Menter Psoriasis Instrument for Identifying Candidate Patients for Systemic Therapy. In: Koo JY, Lebwohl MG, Lee CS, eds: *Mild-to-Moderate Psoriasis*. Informa Healthcare USA, Inc, New York, NY, 2006, pp 9-28.

CHAPTER **5**

Topical Medications for Psoriasis

F our questions a treating physician needs to ask before prescribing topical agents for psoriasis are: Which agent? Which vehicle? Which strength? Which location?

Which Agent?

The most important factor when choosing a topical medication for psoriasis is the choice between steroids and nonsteroids. There are many topical agents to consider, including topical steroids, calcipotriene (Dovonex®), tazarotene (Avage®, Tazorac®), anthralin (Psoriatec™), crude coal tar, salicylic acid, lactic acid, and nonmedicated moisturizers. Our recommendation is to concentrate on using several medications wisely, with a good understanding of appropriate patient candidates, efficacy, side effects, and expected results, rather than mastering all available topical agents. Calcipotriene and topical steroids are two of the most useful topical agents, especially in a primary care setting, and will be examined first. Other, more complicated and perhaps less effective agents, such as tazarotene, anthralin, and tar preparations, will also be discussed.

Lastly, two topical calcineurin inhibitors, tacrolimus (Protopic®) and pimecrolimus (Elidel®) can be used for psoriasis on the face, axilla, and groin. However, these two agents generally are not effective in the treatment of psoriasis other than in the sensitive areas specified above.

Tacrolimus is only available as an ointment in 0.1% or 0.03% concentrations. Pimecrolimus is only available as a cream in a single strength (1%). Both agents tend to work more effectively when applied twice a day rather than once a day, and irritation is the most common side effect. There is a black box warning from the US Food and Drug Administration (FDA) regarding possible cancer risk related to both of these agents, which at this time is based more on theoretical and speculative concerns than on convincing evidence-based data.

Which Vehicle?

Topical medications are available as creams, ointments, foams, gels, lotions, liquid solutions, sprays, and drug-impregnated tapes. The appropriate vehicle to use depends mostly on the location of the psoriasis as well as the patient's preference. Traditionally, it has been taught that thicker vehicles are more potent, more moisturizing, and more effective. With the same active ingredients, ointments are often stronger than creams, which are usually stronger than lotions. However, this is not always true, so it is important to study the efficacy of each individual agent. Moreover, patient preferences often take precedence as long as safety measures are heeded. Patients often appreciate a prescription for both a cream and an ointment of the same agent. Compliance with cream is best in the morning when patients feel more hurried and are thus more likely to forego their treatment. Creams spread across the skin rapidly and easily, are more quickly absorbed than ointments, and do not stain clothing. Ointments are more acceptable in the evenings, when patients have more time for application and are less concerned about the greasiness of the agent interacting with their clothing.

Twice-daily application is critically important for maximal effectiveness of most topical agents (in particular calcipotriene). A patient who is unhappy with a particular vehicle for practical reasons is much less likely to use the medication as directed, and will report a drug as ineffective that may actually be effective if used appropriately. This subsequently limits the available regimens and treatment options, thus forcing the physician to use higher-potency medications. Patients should be routinely encouraged to use these medications as directed so that maximal efficacy can be achieved and patients can rely less on steroids. Ask patients their opinion of their medications and try to work within these preferences to obtain maximal compliance and efficacy.

Consider the location of psoriasis when choosing a treatment vehicle. One area especially sensitive to vehicle choice is the scalp. The scalp presents a particular challenge because hair not only blocks direct application to the plaques, but also will often deter patients from using a cosmetically unsuitable medication despite its effectiveness (Figure 5-1, see color insert). Because of these factors, gels, lotions, liquid solutions, foams, and sprays are the most elegant for treating scalp psoriasis. Creams and ointments are still acceptable, and sometimes more effective, but most patients will prefer to use these at night and wash them out in the morning. One of the most important aspects of treating the scalp is to instruct the patient on appropriate application of a particular medication to ensure that it actually reaches the plaque and not just the hair. Demonstrating the application to the patient in the office with a sample is effective. Finally, be sure that patients understand that the medication must be left on the scalp, rather than washed out like a shampoo. Most treatments can be applied either directly on a dry scalp, or to a damp scalp after towel drying.

Psoriasis symptoms can be another guiding factor in vehicle choice. Patients who complain of dry or itchy skin usually prefer an ointment or cream for added moisturization. Patients with fissures or cracked psoriatic plaques will complain bitterly of stinging pain if alcohol-based agents such as foams or solutions are used. Choose a nonalcohol-based medication for these patients. Gels and foams can be particularly drying and are better suited for patients who dislike the greasiness of creams and ointments, or who have oily skin.

Steroid-impregnated tape (flurandrenolide [Cordran®] tape) can be used when patients have few plaques to treat and are willing to take the time and effort to cut the tape to the appropriate size and apply it to each plaque. This is best done on extremities, where the plaques are thick, scaly, and often resistant to treatment. These areas are also more resistant to skin atrophy that can result under occlusion from steroids.

Which Strength?

Consider the location of psoriasis and disease severity before choosing a strength (Table 5-1). Next, consider the patient. Pediatric patients are more susceptible to skin thinning and should be treated carefully for as short a time as possible when topical steroids are used. Elderly patients are also at higher risk, given their history of sun-damaged and inherently thinner skin. Finally, choose a strength that is conservative, but effective. Steroids are available in seven classes, ranging from over-the-counter hydrocortisone in class 7 to super-potent topical steroids in class 1.

Which Location?

The importance of considering the locations of a patient's psoriasis lies not only in matching it with the most appropriate vehicle, but also in achieving a tolerable side-effect profile, particularly when using topical steroids. The most serious side effects to be aware of when using topical steroids are skin atrophy, including striae or stretch marks, and the risk of adrenal suppression. Atrophic skin appears shiny and thin and is easily traumatized (Figure 5-2, see color insert). The risk of skin atrophy varies according to

Table 5-1: Ranking of Commonly Used Topical Steroids

Group	Brand Name
Class 1	Clobex® lotion
	Clobex® spray
	Clobex® shampoo
	Cormax® cr, ot
	Diprolene® gel, ot
	Psorcon® E™ ot
	Temovate® cr, ot
	Ultravate® cr, ot
Class 2	Cyclocort® ot
	Diprolene® cr
	Diprosone® ot
	Elocon® ot
	Florone® ot
	Halog® cr
	Lidex® cr, gel, ot
	Psorcon® E™ cr
	Topicort® cr
Class 3	Cutivate® ot
	Diprosone® cr
	Halog® ot
	Kenalog® ot
	Lidex® E cr
	Topicort® LP cr
	Valisone® ot
Class 4	Cordran® ot
	Elocon® cr
	Kenalog® cr
	Synalar® ot
	Westcort® ot

cr=cream; ot=ointment

Available Sizes (in grams, unless otherwise specified)	Generic Name
1 oz, 2 oz	Clobetasol propionate
2 oz, 4.25 oz	Clobetasol propionate
4 oz	Clobetasol propionate
15, 30, 45	Clobetasol propionate
15, 45	Betamethasone dipropionate
15, 30, 60	Diflorasone diacetate
15, 30, 45, 60	Clobetasol propionate
15, 50	Halobetasol propionate
15, 30, 60	Amcinonide
15, 45	Betamethasone dipropionate
15, 45	Betamethasone dipropionate
15, 45	Mometasone furoate
15, 30, 60	Diflorasone diacetate
15, 30, 60, 240	Halcinonide
15, 30, 60, 120	Fluocinonide
15, 30, 60	Diflorasone diacetate
15, 60, 4 oz	Desoximetasone
115, 30, 60	Fluticasone propionate
15, 45	Betamethasone dipropionate
15, 30, 60, 240	Halcinonide
15, 20, 60, 80	Triamcinolone acetonide
15, 30, 60, 120	Fluocinonide
15, 60	Desoximetasone
15, 45	Betamethasone valerate
15, 30, 60	Flurandrenolide
15, 45	Mometasone furoate
15, 60, 80	Triamcinolone acetonide
15, 30, 60	Fluocinolone acetonide
15, 45, 60	Hydrocortisone valerate

(continued on next page)

Table 5-1: Ranking of Commonly Used Topical Steroids (continued)

Group	Brand Name
Class 5	Cordran® cr
	Cutivate® cr
	Dermatop® cr
	Locoid® cr
	Synalar® cr
	Valisone® cr
	Westcort® cr
Class 6	Capex® shampoo
	DesOwen® lotion
	DesOwen® cr
	DesOwen® ot
	Aclovate® cr, ot
	Synalar® cr
	Synalar® solution
	Tridesilon® cr, ot
Class 7	Hydrocortisone 2.5%
	Hydrocortisone 1%

cr=cream; ot=ointment; OTC=over the counter

the strength of topical steroid used, the anatomic location to which it is applied, and the length of time the agent is used. On nonsensitive skin, twice-daily use of a topical steroid applied focally (ie, only to the psoriatic plaques and not to unaffected skin) poses little risk of skin atrophy within 2 weeks, even with a high-strength steroid. However, after 2 weeks, the risk of skin atrophy depends on many factors, including individual variations in susceptibility among patients. Susceptibility is unpredictable; even the most

Available Sizes (in grams, unless otherwise specified)	Generic Name
15, 30, 60	Flurandrenolide
15, 30, 60	Fluticasone propionate
15, 60	Prednicarbate
15, 45	Hydrocortisone butyrate
15, 30, 60	Fluocinolone acetonide
15, 45	Betamethasone valerate
15, 45, 60	Hydrocortisone valerate
4 oz	Fluocinolone acetonide
2 oz, 4 oz	Desonide
15, 60, 90	Desonide
15, 60	Desonide
15, 30, 60	Alclometasone dipropionate
15, 30, 60	Fluocinolone acetonide
20 mL, 60 mL	Fluocinolone acetonide
15, 60	Desonide
30, 60	Hydrocortisone
OTC	Hydrocortisone

experienced dermatologist cannot differentiate a susceptible patient from a resistant patient just by clinical examination. Therefore, particularly in a primary care setting, it is best to limit super-potent topical steroid use to the FDA-recommended guideline of 2 weeks continuously or less, and limit lower-strength topical steroids to the shortest possible time needed to gain control of psoriasis. After that, it is preferable to switch to a nonsteroid (ie, calcipotriene) for long-term maintenance.

Steroid-sensitive locations that need special consideration include the face, axilla, pannus skin folds, inner thighs, and groin. These are high-risk areas because they tend to have thinner skin and, in the case of the axilla, groin, and inframammary and abdominal pannus skin folds, create a natural occlusion, which can increase topical potency 10 to 100 times. This makes the area more susceptible to adverse side effects, especially steroid-induced atrophy, striae, telangiectasias, and erythema.

Patients are surprised and disappointed to develop these symptoms if they were inadequately counseled on appropriate use and potential side effects of topical steroids. Physicians are equally distressed because this is one of the most common reasons for dermatologic lawsuits. Striae are usually the most distressing adverse reaction because of their unsightliness and irreversibility (Figure 5-3, see color insert).

If steroids must be used in high-risk areas, physicians may first try those from classes 5, 6, or 7. Topical steroids from class 4 are usually the highest potency acceptable for use in steroid-sensitive areas. Use should be limited over time with the intent of transitioning patients to other, safer topical agents. One pitfall in primary care dermatology is that patients are often instructed appropriately on limiting their steroid use, but then are not given a transition or tapering regimen to follow. This leaves many patients in the trap of treating their disease for 2 weeks and achieving some satisfying results, and then abruptly discontinuing treatment only to see the disease flare again. This vacillating regimen is both frustrating and unproductive, and can be eliminated by the use of sequential therapy (see Chapter 9).

Steroids should also be used carefully on the face. Facial skin is thin, sensitive, and at higher risk for perioral dermatitis, acne, folliculitis, rosacea, hypertrichosis, and hypopigmentation. Again, patients are less tolerant of these side effects because of the cosmetic sensitivity of the area. They should be treated cautiously after adequate counseling. The risk of adverse side effects, however, should be balanced with the severity of disease. If the patient's psoriasis is disfiguring and distressing because of its location, it is worth treating more aggressively with close supervision to improve the patient's quality of life (QOL).

Optimal Use of Topical Steroids for Psoriasis

Psoriasis is thought to be only moderately responsive to topical steroids. Therefore, to obtain an adequate response, the physician needs to use a stronger steroid than what is typically used when treating other common, chronic inflammatory conditions such as eczema or seborrheic dermatitis.

Topical steroid use in psoriasis is also well known to be associated with tachyphylaxis, a phenomenon in which the drugs initially work well, but efficacy gradually diminishes with continuous use. In time, topical steroids may become totally useless. To regain effectiveness, the physician needs to increase steroid potency or give the patient a 'steroid holiday' lasting several months. This drawback has led to the development of intermittent treatment, or pulse therapy, whereby patients use nonsteroid medications such as calcipotriene throughout the week, and steroids only on weekends (see Chapter 9). This approach can be followed long term even with high-potency steroids as long as patients are clinically monitored for side effects.

Steroid strengths typically used for psoriasis range from midstrength agents such as triamcinolone (Kenalog®) 0.1% cream or 0.1% ointment, which are class 4 and 3 respectively, to high-strength agents such as fluocinonide ointment (Lidex®), which is class 2, or mometasone cream or ointment (Elocon®), which is class 4 as a cream or lotion and class 2 as an ointment. Class 1, or super-potent topical steroids such as diflorasone (Psorcon® E™ ointment), betamethasone dipropionate (Diprolene® gel or ointment), clobetasol (Temovate® cream or ointment), or halobetasol (Ultravate® cream or ointment), are the highest-strength steroids available and are often needed for thick, scaly psoriasis. Topical steroids weaker than midstrength generally are not adequately effective for plaque-type psoriasis, especially in nonsensitive areas such as the extremities, where plaques tend to be more resistant.

Physicians should use the lowest possible steroid strength that the patient feels is adequate and the physician believes to be safe. The FDA recommends that class 1 steroids such as clobetasol or halobetasol be used for no more than 2 to 4 weeks at a time (depending on the formulation) and definitely not in sensitive areas, to avoid skin atrophy and adrenal suppression. Longer use requires closer supervision. Whenever topical steroids must be discontinued, they should be tapered off rather than abruptly stopped because abrupt discontinuation may lead to a rebound phenomenon. In this rare phenomenon, psoriasis suddenly becomes even more inflamed than at pretreatment baseline after sudden discontinuation of the steroid, despite replacement with a nonsteroid agent such as calcipotriene.

The amount of class 1 steroid applied each week should also be limited to avoid risk of adrenal suppression. Adrenal suppression may occur with any of the midstrength to super-potent topical steroids. Patients at higher risk include infants and children who have a high skin surface-to-body mass ratio and patients with extensive psoriasis who use large quantities of the drug. For super-potent topical steroids, adult patients should use no more than 2 oz (ie, 50 to 60 g)/week.

Clobetasol in spray formulation (Clobex® spray) is available in the United States. This formulation has impressive efficacy and rapid onset of action. In clinical trials, approximately 70% of the patients were rated as clear or almost clear by the fourth week of treatment using clobetasol spray twice a day. Because this agent is a spray, it can be used to treat psoriasis when larger skin surfaces are involved, in addition to therapy for mild-to-moderate localized psoriasis. Clobetasol spray can also be used to enhance the efficacy of biologic agents. Biologic agents are protein-like material composed of amino acid sequences targeted to interfere with the pathogenesis of psoriasis. Alefacept (Amevive®), efalizumab (Raptiva®), and etanercept (Enbrel®) are examples of biologic agents. Although biologic agents generally have better safety profiles than the prebiologic systemic agents such as cyclosporine (Gengraf®, Neoral®, Sandimmune®) or methotrexate (Trexall™), the overall efficacy and the onset of action can be lower and slower than some prebiologic agents. Clobetasol spray can be used to speed up the onset of action for patients who started on biologic agents. It can also be used to compensate for 'step-down deterioration' sometimes seen with etanercept when the dosage is cut in half after the initial 3 months of therapy. Lastly, even if a patient is stable on a biologic agent, he or she can have occasional flare-ups ('hiccups'), which can often be controlled with the time-limited use of clobetasol spray.

In summary, topical steroids are best suited for a 'quick-fix' or rapid improvement of psoriasis when the patient first presents.

Calcipotriene (Dovonex®) and Calcipotriene/ Betamethasone Dipropionate (Taclonex®) Ointments

Most skin cells possess a nuclear receptor for vitamin D, which has been shown to be responsible for decreasing cellular proliferation and increasing cellular differentiation. For these reasons, vitamin D can be helpful for battling psoriasis. Original trials of oral vitamin D for psoriasis resulted in elevated calcium levels. Calcipotriene is a topical vitamin D analogue modified to minimize the systemic side effects affecting calcium levels. It is not only the first elegant nonsteroidal alternative for the treatment of psoriasis, but is also the most prescribed single agent for psoriasis treatment worldwide.

One of the most important features of calcipotriene that makes it an excellent agent for primary care physicians as well as for dermatologists is its safety profile. Calcipotriene is steroid-free, and thus free from steroid side effects such as skin thinning, striae formation, and adrenal suppression. The primary adverse side effect of calcipotriene is lesional and perilesional (around the lesion) irritation. Irritation from calcipotriene usually presents with a red ring of inflamed skin surrounding the treated lesions (Figure 5-4, see color insert). Patients report a mild stinging or burning sensation. This is usually transient, and patients quickly become accustomed to it. In clinical trials, only one of 25 research subjects had to discontinue treatment because of skin irritation from calcipotriene. The irritation is usually more pronounced on the face and occluded parts of the body such as axilla and groin. It appears to depend largely on the penetration of calcipotriene through the skin. The skin-to-skin occlusion inherent in the axilla and groin enhances penetration of calcipotriene, which is thought to account for the increased rate of irritation in these areas. Calcipotriene also is lipophilic and more readily absorbed by skin containing oily sebaceous glands, such as the face, which also helps explain why it tends to be more irritating on the face.

Irritation from calcipotriene does not necessarily preclude its use; instead, it signifies the need to decrease this agent's skin penetration by using smaller amounts less frequently (eg, once a day or every other day instead of twice a day). Once this regimen is tolerated, the frequency and dose can again be increased carefully. Diluting calcipotriene is another method of reducing potency and thereby reducing irritation. Calcipotriene ointment can be combined easily with pure petrolatum jelly. In rare patients, calcipotriene may cause excessive peeling and apparent expansion of erythema beyond the original border of the psoriasis. If this peculiar perilesional peeling occurs, and if the sensation is not bothersome, it is best to reassure the patient and encourage continued use of calcipotriene until everything, including the expanded erythematous or peeling area, resolves. Another strategy used by most clinicians at the initiation of therapy is combining calcipotriene with a topical steroid. The risk of developing irritation with calcipotriene is greatly reduced when it is used in conjunction with a topical steroid (see Chapter 9).

The systemic adverse side effect to be aware of when using calcipotriene is hypercalcemia. Hypercalcemia has been reported only in rare instances when a patient has used large amounts of this medication on the body. A good guideline to follow is to limit total weekly use of calcipotriene in all formulations (ie, cream, ointment, solution) to 100 to 120 g/week.

Twice-daily application of calcipotriene ointment has been shown in two randomized, double-blind, multicenter studies to be more effective than the use of high-strength topical steroid ointment (ie, fluocinonide) twice daily. However, this result was seen only if the patient used calcipotriene consistently twice a day, every day. In this study, tubes of calcipotriene were weighed after the patients used them, to assure compliance with the twice-daily regimen. If subjects were noncompliant, they were withdrawn from the study. These stringent criteria probably had much to do with the success of the medication. The efficacy of once-daily calcipotriene is approximately half that of twice-daily use during the first month of use, while the efficacy of fluocinonide used once a day is only mildly inferior than twice a day.

Patients need to be well educated when they are given a prescription for calcipotriene. If the patient is to use calcipotriene as monotherapy, it is critical to communicate the importance of using it twice a day and warn of possible skin irritation. In clinical practice, it is difficult to find patients who actually comply with the twice-daily recommended usage. To maximize the chance that a patient will use it this way, it is best to prescribe calcipotriene cream as well as ointment so the patient can use the more elegant but slightly less effective cream in the morning, and more effective but less elegant ointment formulation at night.

Because many patients find time to apply topical medications only once a day, which may lead to slow onset of action and relative dissatisfaction, most dermatologists in the United States use calcipotriene sequentially with a topical steroid, or tazarotene, or both (see Chapter 9). Calcipotriene can be used with many other topical regimens; however, this must be done carefully because calcipotriene is quickly inactivated by acid pH. Therefore, it cannot be used with salicylic acid, lactic acid, or ammonium lactate lotion unless application times are separated by at least 2 hours. When combined with phototherapy, calcipotriene should be applied a minimum of 2 hours before light treatment to prevent inactivation by the ultraviolet A (UVA) wavelengths and rare burning sensations from ultraviolet B (UVB) wavelengths. Combining calcipotriene with other treatment offers not only greater improvement in disease resolution, but also, in the case of topical steroids, a reduction of side effects. The interaction is synergistic: topical steroids limit the risk of skin irritation by calcipotriene, and calcipotriene prevents skin atrophy by the steroid.

A combination ointment for psoriasis involving calcipotriene and betamethasone dipropionate (Taclonex®) recently became available in the United States. It is important to note that the betamethasone dipropionate component of this combination agent is roughly equivalent to high strength rather than super-potent topical steroids. This agent works just as well once a day as twice a day. The skin irritation rate of the calcipotriene/betamethasone dipropionate combination is much less than calcipotriene ointment used alone. In various clinical trials involving >2,000 patients, the calcipotriene/betamethasone dipropionate combination was noted to decrease the average Psoriasis Area and Severity Index (PASI) by 50% to 70% within the first 3 weeks. Moreover, because this agent works well once a day, patients can cover twice the area with the same amount of medication, time, and effort compared with other topical antipsoriasis agents, which usually require twice-daily application to achieve maximum efficacy. Because the topical steroid component of this medication is only high strength rather than super potent, it is feasible to use this agent both for initial clearing (the FDA allows the daily use of this combination agent for up to 1 month) and for long-term maintenance where it is used only 'as needed' or on the weekends. Lastly, compliance with this combination medication is expected to be much better than with the traditional topical agents because of once-a-day dosing and the absence of heightened concerns regarding side effects that are typically associated with the use of super-potent topical steroids.

Other Topical Agents

Other topical agents that may be less effective, require extra caution, or involve special instructions are described below. Potential problems can result because they may be messier or more difficult to use because of their side effect profiles. However, with appropriate knowledge and training, they can be excellent resources when treating psoriasis while avoiding the dangers of excessive reliance on topical steroids.

Tazarotene

Tazarotene is a topical retinoid (modified vitamin A) that is much more powerful than tretinoin (Retin-A®). It was first approved for plaque-type psoriasis in the United States in 1997, and is now also approved for acne and fine-wrinkle reduction. It is available in a cream in 0.05% and 0.1% strengths and a gel in 0.05% and 0.1% strengths. The gel tends to be more elegant, spread more rapidly, and absorb more quickly, making it good for large surfaces as well as for the scalp. The cream is more moisturizing, and, therefore, more appropriate for nonscalp application.

Tazarotene can be effective as a single agent used once daily, but is often used in combination with other treatments, both topical and systemic, to augment therapy and to minimize irritation. Patients who use tazarotene as a monotherapy should apply the medication to the plaques once daily in the evenings, taking care to avoid the surrounding skin.

The most frequently reported side effects of tazarotene are similar to and more commonly reported than those of calcipotriene, including lesional and perilesional irritation, burning, stinging, itching, and redness. Many patients find tazarotene irritating. These patients should be placed on the lower strength. A second option is to decrease the frequency of application to every other day or every third day.

Although tazarotene is effective when used alone, most dermatologists combine it with another agent, either topical or systemic. A recent study showed that once-daily tazarotene in combination with twice-daily calcipotriene is as effective as clobetasol ointment, a class 1 steroid, applied twice daily. Although calcipotriene is a fragile molecule, it can be safely combined with this agent and even used simultaneously by mixing equal parts of one drug with the other and applying the mixture. Mixing cream with cream works best for this, but gel can also be blended in the palm of the patient's hand just before application. Some patients prefer to apply gel first, allow time for its rapid absorption, and then apply cream or ointment over it.

Tazarotene is also a good drug to combine with topical steroids. Efficacy and side-effect profiles of both drugs are better when used in combination. Similar to their use in quelling calcipotriene irritation, topical steroids can help reduce tazarotene irritation. The combination is synergistic in that the skin atrophy resulting from steroid use is thought to be diminished by both calcipotriene and tazarotene. Finally, as reviewed in Chapter 9, all three agents can be successfully and simultaneously combined for maximally effective topical therapy.

A final note to remember about tazarotene when prescribing it in the United States is that it is pregnancy Category X. Although pregnancy data is incomplete and it is considered Category C in Europe, caution should be taken when using this drug in women of child-bearing age based on the risk associated with oral retinoids. Patients should be counseled, have a pregnancy test before starting therapy, and use adequate contraception during treatment.

Anthralin

Due to its moderate efficacy, risk of irritation, and overall messiness, anthralin is one of the less commonly used agents in the United States. It is less effective than twice-daily calcipotriene, but can still be a useful agent in some patients who do not respond to calcipotriene or tazarotene. Most commonly, it is used in a day-care setting as described by the Ingram regimen, using UVB phototherapy followed by all day application of anthralin. Anthralin can also be used at home by motivated patients who fail or do not tolerate other topical treatments or who need to avoid steroids. It can be compounded by an experienced and willing pharmacist in strengths up to 10%, but can often be difficult to find, and must be used with caution.

One disadvantage of anthralin treatment to warn patients about is the inevitable purplish, brownish staining of clothing, porcelain, and skin (Figure 5-5, see color insert). A newer formulation, 1% anthralin, is formulated with a temperature-sensitive vehicle that releases active medication when applied to skin. It shows comparable efficacy with less staining, especially if cool water without soap is used to wash it off. Most patients are willing to tolerate these nuisances to alleviate their symptoms and can be reassured that skin staining disappears several weeks after discontinuing treatment. The most important adverse side effect is skin irritation, usually occurring 3 days after the first application (Figure 5-6, see color insert). This mostly occurs on uninvolved skin, so patients should try to apply the thick paste with a Popsicle stick only to the plaques. Some overlap onto normal surrounding skin is unavoidable, but this often fades with continued use (Figure 5-7, see color insert).

Short-contact therapy remains the most efficacious way to treat patients who are irritated by the medication.

Anthralin is preferentially absorbed by psoriatic plaques, and most of the absorption occurs within the first hour of application. Therefore, applying the medication for 30 minutes to 1 hour before bathing reduces the risk of irritation as well as staining, while maintaining efficacy. Patients should follow with a moisturizing emollient. Phototherapy as well as other topical or oral treatments can be used in combination with anthralin for maximal efficacy.

Coal-Tar Preparations

Coal tar is a mixture of at least 10,000 components, most of which have not been identified. It comes from the distillation of coal in the absence of oxygen. Crude coal tar in combination with phototherapy in a day-care setting is still the most effective treatment available for moderate-to-severe psoriasis since it was first described by Goeckerman in 1925. Coal-tar preparations have some of the longest track records for face usage in actual patients. They can be applied to the entire body on both normal and abnormal skin. Tar products are available in many different formulations and strengths. Getting a good history from the patient will allow the physician to tailor the regimen to the type and location of psoriasis, and to any personal specifications the patient may have. As with anthralin, patients may need to find a pharmacy willing to compound the medication. Additionally, patients can now order some liquid tars directly from Summers Laboratories (Cutar Emulsion® lotion/bath solution 7.5% and Tarsum shampoo/gel® 10% [Table 5-2]).

'Brown tar' is called liquor carbonis detergens (LCD) and can be made in concentrations of up to 20% blended in multiple different vehicles. It is a weak formulation and, therefore, should be prescribed in the higher strength, unless the patient requests otherwise. It can be applied to the skin as a leave-on moisturizer multiple times per day, used in bath water for tar soaks, or used to saturate the scalp under shower-cap occlusion. Patients can achieve added benefit by applying the medication in the evening

Table 5-2: Commonly Used Tar Preparations

'Brown Tar'*

5% LCD	In Nutraderm® lotion
10% LCD	In Nutraderm® lotion
20% LCD	In Nutraderm® lotion

*The above formulations can also be mixed in non-ionic base cream, Aquaphor® ointment, or petrolatum or with triamcinolone lotion, cream, or ointment. Other formulations are available on request.

'Black Tar'**

2% crude coal tar	In petrolatum (ointment)
5% crude coal tar	In petrolatum (ointment)
10% crude coal tar	In petrolatum (ointment)
2% crude coal tar	In nonionic base (cream)

**Each of the above formulations can also be mixed with any of the following: 2%, 5%, or 10% salicylic acid, or 2%, 5%, or 10% lactic acid. Other formulations are available on request.

LCD=liquor carbonis detergens

and occluding it with plastic wrap for increased potency and effectiveness.

'Black tar' is a thick, crude coal-tar product in petrolatum base that can be formulated in 2%, 5%, and 10% strengths. It is primarily used in day-care settings (see Chapter 8), but patients who do not mind the inconvenience can achieve success with home use. They should be encouraged to apply the medication in a downward motion in line with the growth of their hair follicles to decrease the risk of developing folliculitis. Plastic wrap can be used to occlude the tar and reduce soaking into clothing. The tar should be left on for at least 4 hours for maximum efficacy, and many patients complete this regimen at night while sleeping. Mineral oil application followed by bathing and shampooing should be used to remove the medication.

Messiness is one major obstacle when using tar. Old pajamas and bedclothes should be used during this treatment. Side effects of tar products include skin irritation, folliculitis, photosensitivity, and exacerbation of pustular psoriasis. Compared with other psoriasis treatments, tar remains one of the safest. In response to a California lawsuit, the FDA ruled that there is no convincing evidence of carcinogenic risk with human therapeutic use of coal tar in concentration up to 5%.

Salicylic Acid

Keratolytics act to remove excess scale and hyperkeratosis associated with psoriasis. They are available in many different vehicles in strengths ranging from 2% to 20%. Keratolytics can be used on scaly patches on the body as well as on thick, adherent scalp psoriasis. These medications are functional only as 'descaling' agents. They do not affect erythema or induration, and therefore should be used in combination with other topical agents. Patients and Goeckerman day-care centers often mix keratolytics with tar products. One agent that should not be used simultaneously with acidic products is calcipotriene. Calcipotriene is a fragile molecule easily destroyed by acidic pH. However, the two agents can be used together as long as application is separated by at least 2 hours. Salicylic acid is the most commonly used keratolytic agent and is commercially available over the counter as 6% Keralyt® gel. The gel formulation makes it a convenient, easily applied scalp therapy. An excellent regimen using Keralyt® gel is described in Table 5-3.

Table 5-3: Maximal Scalp Treatment Using Keralyt® Gel and LCD

At bedtime:

- Apply Keralyt® gel to scaly areas of scalp.
- Apply 20% liquid carbonis detergens (LCD), using squeeze bottle with tip applicator, to entire scalp by parting hair in 0.5 inch sections and massaging medication in with fingers.
- Cover with shower cap. Place stocking cap or cut thigh section of ladies' nylon stocking over shower cap for better occlusion throughout the night.

In the morning:

- During the morning shower, gently massage scales and medication out of hair with Neutrogena® T/Gel® Shampoo Extra Strength.
- Towel dry hair after showering.
- Apply any combination of tazarotene gel, calcipotriene scalp solution, and steroid solution or foam to damp scalp, taking care to apply medication directly to scalp rather than hair.
- Style hair as usual.
- In the evening, several hours before starting the regimen again, apply second dose of calcipotriene scalp solution and/or topical steroid to achieve twice-daily application.

LCD=liquor carbonis detergens

Salicylic acid can produce local irritation and erythema, especially on normal skin surrounding the psoriatic plaques. In addition, indiscriminate use can lead to excessive systemic absorption, causing salicylism. Symptoms of salicylism include nausea, tinnitus, and hyperventilation. Systemic absorption of salicylic acid can also inhibit gluconeogenesis and lead to hypoglycemia in diabetics. Other agents such as lactic acid should be used for this population.

Selected Readings

Ashton RE, Lowe NJ: Anthralin therapy of psoriasis. In: Lowe NJ, ed: *Practical Psoriasis Therapy,* 2nd ed. St. Louis, MO, Mosby-Year Book, 1993, pp 59-71.

Bowman PH, Maloney JE, Koo JY: Combination of calcipotriene (Dovonex) ointment and tazarotene (Tazorac) gel versus clobetasol ointment in the treatment of plaque psoriasis: a pilot study. *J Am Acad Dermatol* 2002;46:907-913.

Bruce S, Epinette WW, Funicella T, et al: Comparative study of calcipotriene (MC903) ointment and fluocinonide ointment in the treatment of psoriasis. *J Am Acad Dermatol* 1994;31:755-759.

Callis KP, Krueger GG: Topical agents in the treatment of moderate-to-severe psoriasis. In: Weinstein GD, Gottlieb AB, eds: *Therapy of Moderate-to-Severe Psoriasis*, 2nd ed. New York, NY, Marcel Dekker, 2003, pp 29-51.

Christophers E, Mroweitz U: Psoriasis. In: Fitzpatrick TB, Freedberg IM, Eisen AZ, et al, eds: *Dermatology in General Medicine,* 5th ed. New York, NY, McGraw-Hill, 1999, pp 495-533.

Cornell RC, Stoughton RB: Topical steroids. In: Lowe NJ, ed: *Practical Psoriasis Therapy,* 2nd ed. St. Louis, MO, Mosby-Year Book, 1993, pp 33-43.

Goeckerman WH: The treatment of psoriasis. *Northwest Med* 1981;24:229-231.

Gribetz C, Ling M, Lebwohl M, et al: Pimecrolimus cream 1% in the treatment of intertriginous psoriasis: a double-blind, randomized study. *J Am Acad Dermatol* 2004;51:731-738.

Hecker DJ, Lebwohl M: Clinical experience with vitamin D analogues. In: Roenigk HH, Maibach HI, eds: *Psoriasis,* 3rd ed. New York, NY, Marcel Dekker, 1998, pp 507-510.

Koo J, Siebenlist J, et al: Vitamin D analogues in the treatment of psoriasis. In: Roenigk HH, Maibach HI, eds: *Psoriasis,* 3rd ed. New York, NY, Marcel Dekker, 1998, pp 497-506.

Koo JY, Lebwohl MG, Lee CS, eds: *Mild-to-Moderate Psoriasis.* Informa Healthcare USA, Inc, New York, NY, 2006.

Kraft S, Maibach HI, et al: Dithranol (Anthralin). In: Roenigk HH, Maibach HI, eds: *Psoriasis,* 3rd ed. New York, NY, Marcel Dekker, 1998, pp 435-452.

Kragballe K, Austad J, Barnes L, et al: Efficacy results of a 52-week, randomised, double-blind, safety study of a calcipotriol/betamethasone dipropionate two-compound product (Daivobet/Dovobet/Taclonex) in the treatment of psoriasis vulgaris. *Dermatology* 2006;213:319-326.

Kragballe K, van de Kerkhof PC: Consistency of data in six phase III clinical studies of a two-compound product containing calcipotriol and betamethasone dipropionate ointment for the treatment of psoriasis. *J Eur Acad Dermatol Venereol* 2006;20:39-44.

Lebwohl M, Freeman AK, Chapman MS, et al: Tacrolimus ointment is effective for facial and intertriginous psoriasis. *J Am Acad Dermatol* 2004;51:723-730.

Lowe NJ: Tars, keratolytics, and emollients. In: Lowe NJ, ed: *Practical Psoriasis Therapy,* 2nd ed. St. Louis, MO, Mosby-Year Book, 1993, pp 45-57.

Ranking of topical steroids. Galderma Laboratories Inc, Fort Worth, TX, 1999.

Steele JA, Choi C, Kwong PC: Topical tacrolimus in the treatment of inverse psoriasis in children. *J Am Acad Dermatol* 2005;53:713-716.

CHAPTER **6**

Phototherapy

P hototherapy, or the repeated use of ultraviolet light to treat skin disease, is one of the oldest known treatments for psoriasis. It is effective for generalized psoriasis as well as for severe hand and foot psoriasis. Patients can receive treatment either in their dermatologist's office in an outpatient setting or, in some cases, in the comfort and convenience of their own homes. Phototherapy can be accomplished in a standup booth, in front of a standing light panel, with single panels for hands or feet only, or with handheld wands (Figure 6-1, see color insert). The three most common types of phototherapy use ultraviolet A (UVA) wavelengths, ultraviolet B (UVB) wavelengths, or a focused spectrum of UVB called narrow-band UVB (Table 6-1). Examining the methods and principles of phototherapy is beyond the scope of this text. Only general facts will be covered here.

UVB phototherapy includes wavelengths between 290 and 320 nm on the electromagnetic spectrum. Because of its extensive use during the past century and its long track record of safety and efficacy, UVB phototherapy continues to enjoy widespread use. The versatility of UVB adds to its attractiveness. It can be combined with almost any other treatment modality, including topical, oral, and biologic, for greater efficacy. UVB phototherapy is usually reserved to treat psoriasis that is unresponsive to topical medications or too widespread to make twice-daily topical application a feasible option.

If a patient has >10% of their total body surface area involved (1% is approximately equal to the surface area

Table 6-1: Types of Phototherapy

Phototherapy	Procedure
• UVB	290-320 nm
• Narrow-band UVB	311-312 nm
• Oral PUVA	320-400 nm with oral psoralen
• Soak PUVA (or bath-PUVA)	320-400 nm with 30 min psoralen soak prior to light exposure
• Topical PUVA (or paint-PUVA)	320-400 nm with topical psoralen directly applied to the skin by a 'painting' technique

PUVA=psoralen plus ultraviolet A; UVB=ultraviolet B

of the patient's palm plus fingers and thumb), treatment with topical therapy alone is difficult; the patient is likely to need phototherapy and/or systemic therapy in addition to topical agents.

When initiating phototherapy, patients should be treated three times per week. This regimen can later be tapered and eventually maintained at a low frequency or discontinued altogether, but some busy patients find this schedule difficult. In these cases, home light can be an alternative for a reliable and compliant patient.

Side effects and contraindications to phototherapy include burning and photosensitivity reactions. One logistic disadvantage is the extensive time commitment required for this treatment, in addition to three times a week insurance copayments.

Narrow-band UVB is a newer technique that uses a narrower spectrum of energy thought to be most effective for disease clearance. Increasingly popular in Europe and Australia, narrow-band UVB is catching on in the United States. One reason for its popularity is that it has been shown to be more effective than broadband UVB. While there is insufficient data on the carcinogenicity of narrow-band UVB, a century of data collection has revealed no convincing evidence that therapeutic broadband UVB increases the risk of skin cancer. However, a conservative dermatologist may recommend an alternative treatment for the patient known to be prone to skin cancer.

Psoralen plus UVA (PUVA) uses a photosensitizing medication taken orally or absorbed topically in combination with UVA phototherapy. PUVA penetrates more deeply into the tissue than UVB or narrow-band UVB, is more effective than its UVB counterparts, and provides a longer remission. After 30 years of use, PUVA continues to be one of the best psoriasis treatments available, especially for recalcitrant or widespread cases of psoriasis.

Like UVB, PUVA requires a time commitment at least initially, but can be tapered to a maintenance regimen as infrequent as once per month in patients who achieve a complete remission. Such results can dramatically change the life of a suffering patient. However, PUVA also has its own complications, such as nausea, headaches, dizziness (when taken orally), burning, itching, and photosensitivity. Proven in white patients only, it has been shown that PUVA increases the risk of developing squamous cell skin cancer. Controversy continues about whether it increases the risk of melanoma with long-term use. Thus far, one large-scale study showed an increased risk of melanoma only after 15 years of follow-up, and mainly in those who had at least 250 PUVA treatments. Another large-scale, long-term study showed no increased risk of melanoma with PUVA. Approximately 20 other published studies with smaller cohorts and/or shorter follow-up periods failed to demonstrate increased risk of melanoma. Squamous cell carcinoma and melanomas are relevant issues primarily for fair-skinned individuals or for those patients who have had at least 200 to 250 treatment sessions.

One important point to remember when caring for a patient receiving phototherapy is the interaction of light with other medications. The list of photosensitizing drugs is extensive; common offenders include thiazide diuretics, loop diuretics, antibiotics, antidepressants, and antipsychotics. Use of these medications is not prohibited, but communication about them is essential. Treating physicians and nurses must be aware of photosensitizing medications, especially when they are initiated midtreatment, so that light can be adjusted accordingly to avoid burning patients or precipitating a phototoxic reaction.

Finally, for patients who are unable to carry out phototherapy, heliotherapy may be an option, especially in darker skin types. Heliotherapy is the purposeful, methodical exposure to sunlight or tanning beds. All patients should be instructed on safe methods of exposure.

Selected Readings

Koo JY, Bandow G, et al: The art and practice of UVB phototherapy for the treatment of psoriasis. In: Weinstein GD, Gottlieb AB, eds: *Therapy of Moderate-to-Severe Psoriasis*, 2nd ed. New York, NY, Marcel Dekker, 2003, pp 53-90.

Lindelof B, Sigurgeirsson B, Tegner E, et al: PUVA and cancer risk: the Swedish follow-up study. *Br J Dermatol* 1999;141:108-112.

Morison WL: Systemic and topical PUVA therapy. In: Weinstein GD, Gottlieb AB, eds: *Therapy of Moderate-to-Severe Psoriasis*, 2nd ed. New York, NY, Marcel Dekker, 2003, pp 91-114.

Stern RS, Nichols KT, Vakeva LH: Malignant melanoma in patients treated for psoriasis with methoxsalen (psoralen) and ultraviolet A radiation (PUVA). The PUVA Follow-Up Study. *N Engl J Med* 1997;336:1041-1045.

CHAPTER 7

Oral Agents

Systemic Corticosteroids

Systemic corticosteroids are not indicated for the treatment of psoriasis and should be avoided whenever possible. Although they are effective in improving psoriatic lesions, patients will quickly relapse and can experience severe rebound upon discontinuation. Rebound occurs when patients develop even larger areas of psoriasis than before they began treatment or when the characteristics of their disease change to a more serious form of psoriasis (eg, conversion from plaque-type to erythrodermic or pustular psoriasis). The eruption that occurs after withdrawal from treatment with systemic corticosteroids is often more recalcitrant to treatment than the initial disease. Of course, a patient may require systemic corticosteroids for treatment of a concomitant medical condition (eg, asthma or arthritis exacerbation). Be aware of the potential for psoriasis rebound upon cessation of the medication.

Methotrexate

Methotrexate (Trexall™) was approved by the US Food and Drug Administration (FDA) for use in psoriasis in the early 1970s. Originally, methotrexate was thought to slow the pathologic increase in the rate of cell replication found in psoriatic skin by interfering with DNA synthesis. However, methotrexate most likely acts through an immunosuppressive rather than an antiproliferative mechanism. In addition to improving skin lesions, methotrexate has been shown to be efficacious in the treatment of psoriatic arthritis and nail psoriasis.

Methotrexate should be avoided in patients with renal, hepatic, or hematologic abnormalities. Patients with a history of alcohol abuse should not use methotrexate because hepatotoxicity is associated with long-term exposure to alcohol. In the absence of risk factors for liver disease, a baseline liver biopsy is not necessary before starting methotrexate. In patients with persistently abnormal liver function tests (LFTs) or risk factors for hepatic disease, a pretreatment liver biopsy is required. Methotrexate is teratogenic and Category X, and women should not conceive, nor should men impregnate anyone, while they are taking the drug and for 3 months following the last dose. This medication also carries several black box warnings, including an increased risk of lymphoma and methotrexate-induced pneumonitis.

Before initiating therapy, certain tests including baseline renal function tests, LFTs, and a complete blood count (CBC) should be performed to ensure no contraindications are present. If these laboratory tests are within normal limits, a test dose of 2.5 to 5 mg is typically given to assess tolerability and safety. Laboratory tests should be repeated several days after taking the test dose, and the patient should be asked about any side effects. The most common symptoms reported with the use of methotrexate include nausea, vomiting, malaise, and headache. An antiemetic can be added, if needed. More serious adverse reactions to be aware of are bone marrow suppression, hepatotoxicity, and pneumonitis, which are rare. Additionally, patients can develop acute photosensitivity after starting methotrexate. This is especially relevant in patients undergoing concomitant phototherapy. Light therapy should not be given for 48 to 72 hours after the administration of methotrexate. Generally, the severity of side effects is dose-related, and methotrexate can be titrated to maximize efficacy while minimizing adverse side effects. The usual dose required for good clearing in a nonelderly adult patient is 15 mg/week taken in three divided doses, 12 hours apart; a typical maximum dose of up to 30 mg weekly can be given. Laboratory tests must be repeated every 6 weeks, and the dermatologic standard of care mandates that a liver biopsy be performed after a total cumulative dose of 1.5 g initially, then every 1 to 1.5 g thereafter.

While a dermatologist or rheumatologist will most often be the prescribing and monitoring physician for methotrexate, the primary care physician needs to be aware of potential drug interactions that may occur while caring for the psoriasis patient on methotrexate. Trimethoprim (found in Bactrim™ and Septra®), in combination with methotrexate, can cause severe bone marrow suppression and should never be given concomitantly. Barbiturates, probenecid (Probalan®), phenytoin (Dilantin®, Phenytek®), sulfonamides, and some nonsteroidal anti-inflammatory drugs (NSAIDs) can increase the serum level or half-life of methotrexate through various mechanisms. Table 7-1 lists drugs to avoid when taking methotrexate.

Cyclosporine

Cyclosporine (Gengraf®, Neoral®, Sandimmune®) works in part by inhibiting T-cell production of interleukin-2 (IL-2), a cytokine that plays a key role in activating T cells and propagating the inflammatory cascade. Cyclosporine is usually reserved for patients with severe psoriasis and is especially appropriate for systemically healthy patients who present with erythrodermic psoriasis. At a higher dosage range (ie, 4 to 5 mg/kg/day), the effects of cyclosporine are rapid and dramatic compared with the slower onset of action of other psoriasis treatments. While liver toxicity is the major concern with methotrexate, the kidney is the target organ for toxicity with cyclosporine. Patients need to be closely monitored for the development of nephrotoxicity and hypertension, and cyclosporine should be avoided in patients with baseline renal dysfunction.

Patients who are considered for cyclosporine therapy must be free of serious infection, immunosuppressive states

Table 7-1: Drugs to Avoid When Taking Methotrexate

- Trimethoprim/sulfamethoxazole (TMP/SMX) (Bactrim™, Septra®)
- Aminoglycosides
- Salicylates
- Phenylbutazone
- Sulfonamides
- Probenecid (Probalan®)
- Cephalothin
- Penicillins
- Colchicine
- Nonsteroidal anti-inflammatory drugs (NSAIDs)
- Ethanol
- Pyrimethamine (Daraprim®, Fansidar®)
- Triamterene (Dyrenium®)
- Barbiturates
- Phenytoin (Dilantin®, Phenytek®)
- Retinoids
- Sulfonylureas
- Tetracycline
- Dipyridamole (Aggrenox®, Persantine®)

(eg, human immunodeficiency virus [HIV]), and current signs or a history of malignancy. Malignancies have been reported in transplant patients who have received cyclosporine for an extended period at doses two to three times those used in dermatology. However, studies have failed to show any convincing evidence for an increase in internal cancers, including lymphoma, in psoriasis patients whose treatment with cyclosporine followed dermatologic guidelines. Some data suggests a slight-to-moderate increase in nonmelanoma skin cancer risk, which may primarily be of concern to white people who have had previous exposure to psoralen plus ultraviolet A (PUVA) phototherapy. Cyclosporine should be used cautiously in patients with a long history of treatment with PUVA because they already have an increased risk of developing skin cancer.

Before initiating therapy, two baseline blood pressure readings should be obtained. Additionally, the following laboratory tests must be performed: renal function tests and LFTs with two creatinine measurements at least 24 hours apart, magnesium and potassium levels, a CBC, and a fasting lipid profile. If these results are within normal limits, cyclosporine can be started at a dosage of 3 mg/kg/day and titrated upward by 0.5 to 1 mg/kg/day every month to a maximum of 5 mg/kg/day. However, if the disease is severe and disabling enough, we recommend starting at the maximum dose and tapering downward. Ideal body weight should be used to avoid overdosing in patients who are obese. Laboratory tests and blood pressure should be repeated 2 weeks after the initial dose and every 2 to 6 weeks thereafter. According to FDA guidelines, uninterrupted treatment with cyclosporine can be given for a maximum of only 1 year at a time to minimize the risk of nephrotoxicity; international guidelines extend this to 2 years. Patients need to take a 'drug holiday' of at least 3 to 4 months before restarting the medication.

The development of hypertension or decreased renal function does not mean cyclosporine must be discontinued. If a patient's creatinine increases above baseline by 30% or if the patient's blood pressure elevates above a diastolic of 90 mm Hg, the dose of cyclosporine can be decreased until these values normalize. The dermatologist may need to partner with the primary care physician to help control high blood pressure with antihypertensives. The calcium-channel blockers nifedipine (Adalat® CC, Procardia®,

Procardia® XL) and isradipine (DynaCirc CR®) are the agents of choice in this situation because they do not alter serum levels of cyclosporine, while verapamil (Calan®, Isoptin® SR) and diltiazem (Cardizem®) are not recommended because they can alter serum levels of cyclosporine. The patient who develops hyperlipidemia may also require the use of lipid-lowering agents.

Other side effects encountered with cyclosporine include nausea, headache, hypertrichosis, gingival hyperplasia, and paresthesias. Like those of methotrexate, cyclosporine's side effects are generally reversible and dose-dependent. Cyclosporine is not teratogenic, but it has been associated with low birth weight and premature labor. Drug interactions include certain antibiotics, antifungals, diuretics, H_2-blockers, and oral contraceptives. These drugs may raise levels of cyclosporine, increasing the risk of nephrotoxicity. Grapefruit juice is also known to elevate serum cyclosporine levels. Cyclosporine can reduce the clearance of digoxin (Lanoxin®), lovastatin (Mevacor®), and prednisone. Table 7-2 lists drugs to avoid when taking cyclosporine.

Acitretin

Acitretin (Soriatane®) is a synthetic retinoid that normalizes the hyperproliferative state of psoriatic skin by enhancing the maturation and differentiation of keratinocytes. It has a slow onset of action and does not always clear erythema on its own. For these reasons, it is not optimal for use as a monotherapy. However, it is safe for long-term use with proper supervision and can be used for an unlimited time, provided that no problem develops clinically, radiologically, or with respect to laboratory findings, making it useful for maintenance therapy. It also enhances other modalities of treatment, such as phototherapy, and has no serious drug interactions with other psoriasis treatments (except increasing the risk of hepatotoxicity when used with methotrexate), which makes it a useful choice in combination therapy. High-dose acitretin is especially

Table 7-2: Drugs to Avoid When Taking Cyclosporine

- Ketoconazole (Nizoral®)
- Fluconazole (Diflucan®)
- Itraconazole (Sporanox®)
- Amphotericin B (Abelcet®, AmBisome®, Amphotec®, Fungizone®)
- Gentamicin
- Tobramycin (Tobi®)
- Vancomycin
- TMP/SMX (Bactrim™, Septra®)
- Erythromycin (Ery-Tab®, Erythrocin®)
- Norfloxacin (Noroxin®)
- Cephalosporins
- Doxycycline (Vibramycin®)
- Acyclovir (Zovirax®)
- Oral contraceptives

TMP/SMX=trimethoprim/sulfamethoxazole

efficacious in the treatment of patients with generalized pustular psoriasis. The combination of retinoids with PUVA or ultraviolet B light (UVB), known as re-PUVA or re-UVB, is also the treatment of choice for hand and foot psoriasis, and this combination is used to transition patients off cyclosporine.

Side effects commonly encountered with acitretin can be uncomfortable for patients. These include significant drying of the mucous membranes, such as the lips and eyes,

- Corticosteroids
- Danazol
- Cimetidine (Tagamet®)
- Ranitidine (Zantac®)
- Thiazide diuretics
- Furosemide (Lasix®)
- Warfarin (Coumadin®)
- Diltiazem (Cardizem®)
- Nicardipine (Cardene®)
- Verapamil (Calan®, Isoptin® SR)
- Bromocriptine (Parlodel®)
- Metoclopramide (Reglan®)
- Diclofenac (Cataflam®)
- Melphalan (Alkeran®)

hair loss, headache, myalgia, decreased night vision, and pyogenic granulomas around the nails. Patients often need to be reassured and provided with symptomatic care. More serious adverse reactions can include an elevation of serum triglycerides (Tgs) and cholesterol, although this is usually easy to control with lipid-lowering agents. LFT results can also become abnormally elevated; however, this elevation is often transient, and progression to fibrosis and cirrhosis is extremely rare. A rare side effect of long-term retinoid use is calcification of the ligaments and bony changes in the form of diffuse idiopathic skeletal hyperostosis (DISH) syndrome; however, data are conflicting. Several large, prospective studies failed to show an increased risk of de novo hyperostosis in patients taking acitretin.

Depression is an adverse reaction associated with retinoids and is the subject of much controversy. Only isotretinoin (Accutane®) has been linked to depression and suicide, and this association is debatable because the age group of patients taking isotretinoin (ie, teenagers) has higher rates of depression and suicide at the outset. The extrapolation of this association to other retinoids such as acitretin has not been scientifically substantiated. However, it is sound medicolegal practice to inform the patient of the controversial relationship between depression and retinoids, screen for any mood disorders, and instruct the patient to inform his or her dermatologist about any mood changes. If a mood disturbance occurs, acitretin should be discontinued immediately.

Before initiating therapy, patients must have a baseline CBC, fasting lipid profile, and LFTs performed. If these evaluations are within normal limits, acitretin can be started at a dose of 25 mg/day. The medication should always be taken with food because this significantly increases its absorption. The dose can be titrated upward as tolerated in increments of 10 mg up to a usual maximum of 50 mg/day. Laboratory tests should be repeated 2 weeks after the initial dose or a dose increase, then in 4 weeks, and then again in 8 weeks. Monitoring may be as infrequent as once every 3 months for long-term, low-dose (≤25 mg/day) maintenance therapy. Acitretin is known to enhance the efficacy of UVB and PUVA and decreases the amount of light exposure required to control the disease. In turn, when re-PUVA or re-UVB is used, an acitretin dose of 25 mg/day is usually adequate to achieve good enhancement of phototherapy. Some evidence suggests that systemic retinoid use has a protective effect against the development of skin cancers.

This makes it a more favorable agent to use in patients undergoing long-term phototherapy.

Because acitretin is a Category X drug, women should not conceive while on this drug and for a minimum of 3 years after the last dose. This drug should be avoided in women of childbearing potential, especially those who plan on having children in the near future. Those who are of reproductive age and do not plan on having children should be educated about the teratogenic potential of acitretin and instructed to use two effective forms of birth control during therapy and for a minimum of 3 years posttreatment. They should start acitretin on the second or third day after menses has started and be monitored with regular urine pregnancy tests. When choosing oral contraceptives, it is important to know that acitretin may interfere with the effectiveness of the progestin 'minipill.' Men are unaffected and can be reassured that acitretin will not affect their reproductive potential. Because active metabolites can be present in the blood for up to 3 years posttreatment, patients should also be instructed not to donate blood during therapy and for 3 years afterward.

While acitretin has few drug interactions, several are worth noting. Milk can increase its absorption, and vitamin A can increase its toxicity. Taking tetracycline concomitantly has been associated with an increase in the extremely rare incidence of pseudotumor cerebri. Ethanol can increase the half-life of acitretin in the body and should be avoided during and for up to 2 months after treatment, especially in women.

Hydroxyurea

Like methotrexate, hydroxyurea (Droxia®, Hydrea®) inhibits DNA synthesis and the rapid cell turnover found in psoriasis. Although not FDA-approved for the treatment of psoriasis, hydroxyurea has been used off-label in combination therapy for years. The average dose of hydroxyurea is 1 g taken daily in two divided doses. Because the major toxicity associated with hydroxyurea is hematopoietic,

Table 7-3: Summary of Oral Agents for Psoriasis Treatment

Drug	Dose
Methotrexate (Trexall™)	2.5-5 mg test dose 15-30 mg/wk, divided into 2-3 doses, taken q8-12h within 24 h
Cyclosporine (Gengraf®, Neoral®, Sandimmune®)	3-5 mg/kg/d divided twice daily
Acitretin (Soriatane®)	10-50 mg once daily
Hydroxyurea* (Droxia®, Hydrea®)	1-2 g/d divided twice daily

*Off-label use

CBCs should be performed every 4 to 6 weeks to monitor for potential bone marrow suppression. Mild-to-moderate anemia with macrocytosis often occurs, while the occurrence of leukocytosis and thrombocytopenia is rare. All hematologic parameters usually normalize 6 to 8 weeks after cessation of therapy. Hepatic and renal toxicity, al-

Laboratory Tests	Major Toxicities
CBC	Hepatotoxicity
LFTs	Bone marrow suppression
BUN and creatinine	Teratogenicity
Liver biopsy	GI disturbance
CBC	Nephrotoxicity
LFTs	Hypertension
BUN and creatinine	Hyperlipidemia
Potassium and magnesium	Hypertrichosis
Fasting lipid profile	Paresthesias
CBC	Mucocutaneous changes
LFTs	Hyperlipidemia
Fasting lipid profile	Teratogenicity
Pregnancy test	Hepatotoxicity
	Hyperostosis
CBC	Bone marrow suppression
LFTs	
BUN and creatinine	

BUN= blood urea nitrogen; CBC=complete blood count
GI=gastrointestinal; LFT=liver function test

though unusual, have been reported, so LFTs and kidney function tests should be checked regularly. Cutaneous changes associated with hydroxyurea include generalized hyperpigmentation, alopecia, and leg ulcer development.

Hydroxyurea has a slow onset of action and shows only partial efficacy in most cases. It is often used in combination with other systemic treatments. It can enhance a patient's response to phototherapy and can be used together with agents that have differing side-effect profiles (eg, acitretin). It can be particularly helpful in cases of stubborn hand and foot psoriasis.

Table 7-3 summarizes available oral agents for psoriasis treatment.

Selected Readings

Callen JP, Kulp-Shorten CL, Wolverton SE: Methotrexate. In: Wolverton SE, ed: *Comprehensive Dermatologic Drug Therapy.* Philadelphia, PA, WB Saunders Co, 2001, pp 147-164.

Goldfarb MT, Ellis CN: Clinical use of etretinate and acitretin. In: Roenigk HH, Maibach HI, eds: *Psoriasis*, 3rd ed. New York, NY, Marcel Dekker, 1998, pp 663-670.

Koo JY, Gambla C, Lee J: Cyclosporin for the treatment of psoriasis. In: Roenigk HH, Maibach HI, eds: *Psoriasis*, 3rd ed. New York, NY, Marcel Dekker, 1998, pp 641-658.

Koo JY, Lee CS, Maloney JE: Cyclosporine and related drugs. In: Wolverton SE, ed: *Comprehensive Dermatologic Drug Therapy.* Philadelphia, PA, WB Saunders Co, 2001, pp 205-229.

Lebwohl MG, Feldman SR, Koo JY, et al: *Psoriasis: Treatment Options and Patient Management.* National Psoriasis Foundation, 2002, pp 45-72.

Roenigk HH, Maibach HI: Methotrexate. In: Roenigk HH, Maibach HI, eds: *Psoriasis*, 3rd ed. New York, NY, Marcel Dekker, 1998, pp 609-630.

Smith C, Barker J, Menter MA: *Psoriasis.* Oxford, England, Health Press, 2002, pp 51-56.

Wright S, Gemzik B: Hydroxyurea. In: Roenigk HH, Maibach HI, eds: *Psoriasis*, 3rd ed. New York, NY, Marcel Dekker, 1998, pp 631-636.

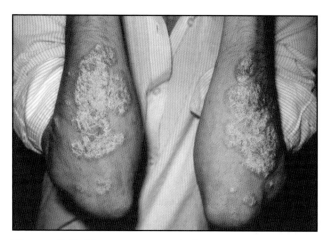

Figure 1-1: Plaque-type psoriasis.

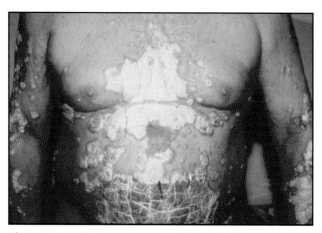

Figure 1-2: Severe, generalized psoriasis.

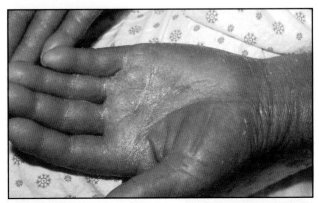

Figure 2-1: Carnauba wax appearance of pityriasis rubra pilaris.

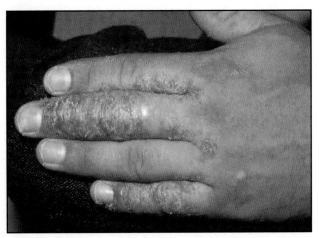

Figure 2-2: Hand eczema.

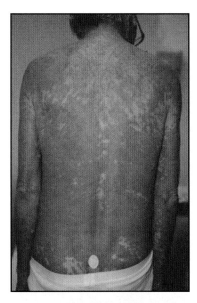

Figure 3-1:
Erythrodermic
psoriasis.

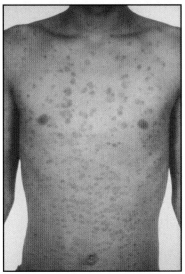

Figure 3-2:
Guttate psoriasis.

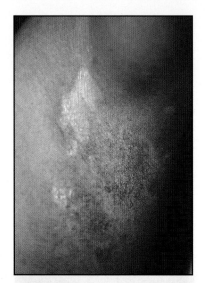

Figure 3-3:
Inverse psoriasis of the axilla.

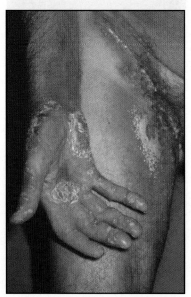

Figure 3-4:
Pustular psoriasis.

I-4

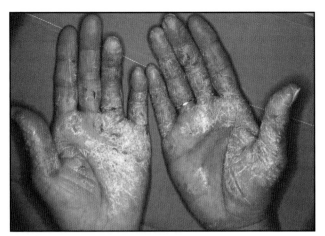

Figure 3-5: Hand psoriasis.

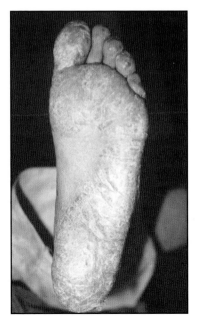

Figure 3-6:
Foot psoriasis.

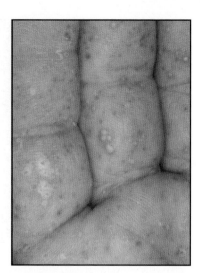

Figure 3-7:
Localized pustular hand psoriasis.

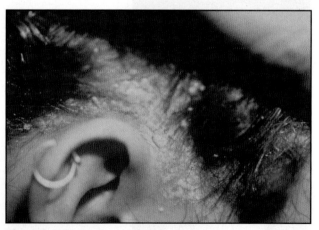

Figure 5-1: Scalp psoriasis.

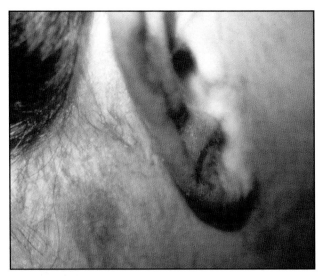

Figure 5-2: Skin atrophy (seen behind the ear) from chronic topical corticosteroid use.

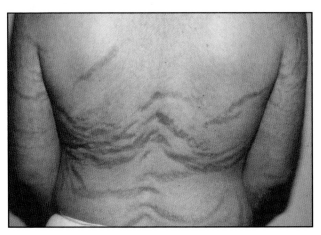

Figure 5-3: Striae from chronic topical corticosteroid use.

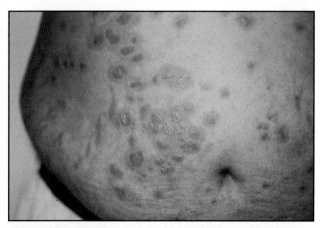

Figure 5-4: Perilesional irritation from calcipotriene.

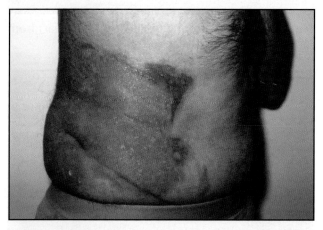

Figure 5-5: Perilesional irritation and pigmentation from anthralin.

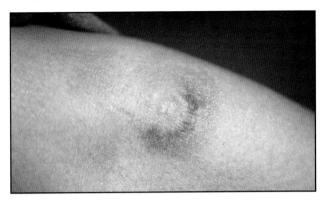

Figure 5-6: Perilesional irritation from anthralin.

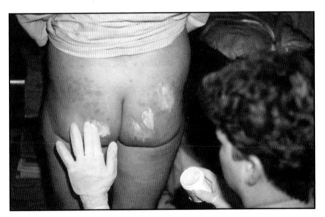

Figure 5-7: Application of anthralin.

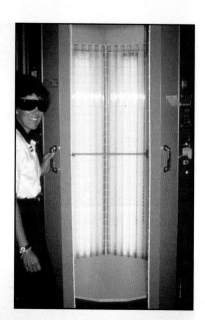

Figure 6-1:
Phototherapy unit.

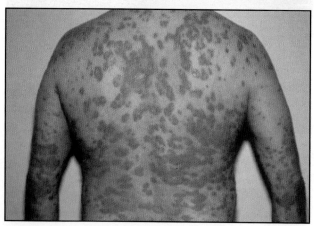

Figure 8-1: Generalized psoriasis before Goeckerman therapy.

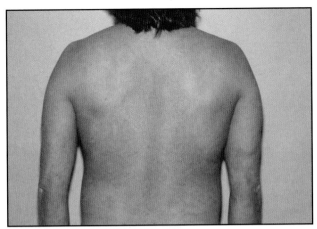

Figure 8-2: Generalized psoriasis after 28 days of Goeckerman therapy.

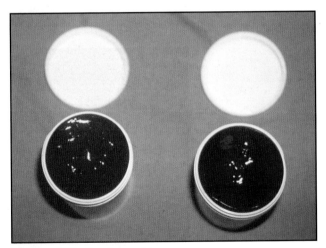

Figure 8-3: Crude coal tar.

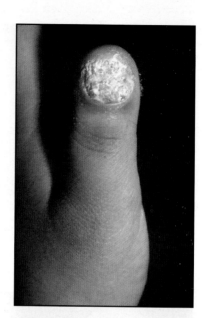

Figure 11-1:
Nail psoriasis.

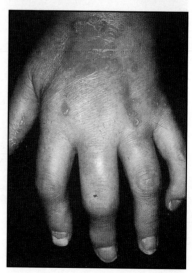

Figure 12-1:
Psoriatic arthritis with boutonniere deformity.

CHAPTER 8

Inpatient (Goeckerman) Therapy

I npatient therapy, also known as Goeckerman therapy, is one of the oldest regimens for treating psoriasis. Despite the excitement generated by newer oral agents and injectable biologics, inpatient therapy remains the fastest, safest, and most effective treatment for moderate-to-severe psoriasis. Data from the University of California San Francisco Psoriasis Treatment Center shows that PASI 75 (≥75% improvement in the Psoriasis Area Severity Index [PASI]) at 3 months with Goeckerman therapy is 100%. Additionally, among published data on average remission times with various psoriasis therapies, Goeckerman therapy offers the longest known remission time (Figures 8-1 and 8-2, see color insert).

Traditionally, Goeckerman therapy took place in an inpatient setting. It was a 24-hour-per-day treatment course until patients were discharged. Because of problems with reimbursement under managed care, and because of the inconvenience to patients, this course has become a day-care procedure in most facilities today. Patients are treated 8 hours/day, 5 days/week, until their disease clears, which usually takes 20 to 30 treatment days. Patients typically begin the day with ultraviolet B (UVB) phototherapy. Following light treatment, crude coal tar in concentrations up to 10% (often with salicylic acid or lactic acid) is applied to the entire body, including normal skin. Intertriginous areas are avoided unless they contain psoriasis. Patients are then wrapped with plastic wrap for occlusive purposes, and dressed in old pajamas or scrubs. After they are fully dressed, their scalp is treated with 20% liquor carbonis detergens (LCD) (see description in Chapter 5) and occluded with a shower cap. Patients can then relax until the afternoon. To remove the tar, they use mineral oil and routine showering. Finally, they apply brown tar (20% LCD in Aquaphor®) before going home and again at bedtime. The most critical detail contributing to the high efficacy of Goeckerman therapy is the use of black crude coal tar rather than refined or diluted tar preparations, which are typically brown or gold in appearance (Figure 8-3, see color insert).

In some patients, psoriasis clears in as little as 2 weeks. More severely affected patients require longer treatments. For these patients, additional therapies can be combined with Goeckerman therapy. Modern use of Goeckerman therapy often includes the original ingredients of UVB phototherapy and black tar supplemented with other modalities, including anthralin (compounded up to 10% in concentration), salicylic acid, lactic acid, calcipotriene (Dovonex®), tazarotene (Avage®, Tazorac®), and even the concurrent use of oral medications such as acitretin (Soriatane®) or biologics to enhance the entire process. Bath-psoralen plus ultraviolet A (PUVA) phototherapy can be added for resistant cases or resistant anatomic locations. Patients who are receiving UVB and PUVA phototherapy together should receive UVB first, before the application of psoralen, to avoid inadvertent exposure to contaminating UVA wavelengths while receiving UVB phototherapy.

In the past, Goeckerman therapy was widely practiced in the United States as the 'gold standard' for psoriasis. With the advent of managed care, there are only a few places capable of conducting traditional Goeckerman therapy. Overseas, this therapy remains an essential treatment option, especially for severe disease.

Selected Readings

Horwitz S: Ultraviolet therapy with coal tars. In: Lowe NJ, ed: *Practical Psoriasis Therapy*, 2nd ed. St. Louis, MO, Mosby-Year Book, 1993, pp 95-113.

Koo J, Lebwohl M: Duration of remission of psoriasis therapies. *J Am Acad Dermatol* 1999;41:51-59.

Koo JY, Lebwohl MG, Lee CS, eds: *Mild-to-Moderate Psoriasis*. Informa Healthcare USA, Inc, New York, NY, 2006.

Lee E, Koo J: Modern modified 'ultra' Goeckerman therapy: a PASI assessment of a very effective therapy for psoriasis resistant to both prebiologic and biologic therapies. *J Dermatolog Treat* 2005; 16:102-107.

CHAPTER **9**

Combination, Rotational, and Sequential Therapies

Optimizing therapy for patients with psoriasis that is resistant to traditional therapies requires balancing many factors, including safety, efficacy, onset of benefit, and duration of response. Because of the complexity of these multiple factors, optimal treatment for most patients is achieved through the use of creative therapeutic strategies, such as combination, rotational, and sequential therapies.

Using two agents that work through different mechanisms of action can maximize therapeutic results by merging the strengths and minimizing the weaknesses of each. For example, an agent with a less favorable side-effect profile and rapid onset of action can be used together with a slower-acting, less toxic agent. The drug used for its speed of action can then be tapered, and the patient maintained on the slower but safer agent. Cyclosporine (Gengraf®, Neoral®, Sandimmune®) works quickly and effectively, but is not suitable for long-term use because of its nephrotoxic potential. Acitretin (Soriatane®) is safer to use for extended periods but has a slow onset of action. Using both agents combines the benefits of rapid clearance with safe maintenance. Another benefit of using multiple agents is that patients can usually achieve the same response on doses of agents used in combination that are much lower than those required when each is used as a monotherapy. A good example of this phenomenon is the use of retinoids with phototherapy. Doses of acitretin and cumulative expos-

Table 9-1: Potential Combinations

Useful Combinations

- Topicals and phototherapy
- Topicals and retinoids
- Topicals and immunomodulators
- Retinoids and phototherapy
- Methotrexate (Trexall™) and phototherapy
- Hydroxyurea (Droxia®, Hydrea®) and phototherapy
- Biologics and phototherapy
- Retinoids and cyclosporine
- Methotrexate and cyclosporine (Gengraf®, Neoral®, Sandimmune®)
- Retinoids and biologics
- Cyclosporine and biologics
- Methotrexate and biologics

Combinations Requiring Caution

- Cyclosporine and phototherapy
- Methotrexate and retinoids
- Any combination of bone marrow suppressants (ie, methotrexate, hydroxyurea, 6-thioguanine)

ure to ultraviolet B (UVB) or psoralen plus ultraviolet A (PUVA) can be reduced when these therapies are used together. Certain combinations are to be avoided, particularly cyclosporine and phototherapy, because of the increased risk of skin cancer with long-term use, especially in white patients. Combining agents that have similar side-effect profiles, such as methotrexate (Trexall™) and hydroxy-urea (Droxia®, Hydrea®), which are both associated with bone marrow suppression, can result in increased toxicity. Methotrexate and acitretin in combination warrants caution because of the additive risks of hepatotoxicity. Table 9-1 lists potential combinations.

Rotational Therapy

Rotational therapy minimizes cumulative toxicity by switching between agents with differing toxicity profiles. Many systemic agents have side effects that are dose-dependent and reversible upon discontinuation of the drug. Therapies such as cyclosporine cannot be used for an extended period on an uninterrupted basis. By switching from one therapeutic regimen to another, the patient is given a 'holiday' from one particular treatment. For example, a patient can be on cyclosporine for 1 year, switched to methotrexate for another year, put on phototherapy for 1 to 2 years, started on a course of alefacept (Amevive®), efalizumab (Raptiva®), or etanercept (Enbrel®), until, finally, cyclosporine is initiated again and the cycle is repeated.

Sequential Therapy

Sequential therapy is a commonly employed strategy in which agents are used in a deliberate sequence to maximize the initial speed of improvement while minimizing long-term toxicity. The three phases of sequential therapy are step 1, the clearing phase; step 2, the transition phase; and step 3, the maintenance phase (Table 9-2).

The classic example of topical sequential therapy involves calcipotriene (Dovonex®) and halobetasol (Ultravate®). Super-potent topical corticosteroids are more efficacious and work more rapidly than calcipotriene. However, long-term use can result in skin atrophy and adrenal suppression. Calcipotriene is effective over time and safe to use long term, but is slower to act and associated with irritation. Using both medications sequentially optimizes the rate and degree of clearance by combining their strengths and allowing them to counteract individual weaknesses. When applied together, there is a synergistic enhancement of efficacy, and improvement can be more rapid than when either agent is used alone. The presence of a steroid decreases the risk of calcipotriene irritation, while maintenance with calcipotriene eliminates the risk of skin atrophy and adrenal suppression that is associated with long-term steroid use. The gradual transition off steroids prevents the rebound that can occur after abrupt discontinuation.

Step 1 consists of using both agents, mixed in a 1:1 ratio and applied twice daily. Once mixed, these agents can begin destroying each other in 48 hours, therefore, it is imperative that the patient mixes them immediately before application. If the patient is compliant with this regimen, clearance can be expected in approximately 1 month. During the transition phase, a gradual tapering of the steroid takes place. Calcipotriene alone is used twice daily on weekdays, while the combination is used twice daily on weekends to 'pulse' the patient with steroids. The patient usually continues step 2 for approximately 1 month, but some resistant cases may require steroid pulse therapy indefinitely (ie, weekday/weekend regimen). If periodically supervised, patients can be safely maintained on step 2 indefinitely since it would be extremely unusual for a patient to develop adrenal suppression or skin atrophy when using topical steroids only 2 days/week. Most patients should begin step 3 as soon as possible, which consists of maintenance with calcipotriene alone, twice daily. If relapse occurs, the patient can be moved back to step 2 or step 1 and then switched to step 3 as control of the disease is attained again.

The same 'rabbit-to-turtle' model of sequential therapy can be used for systemic agents to maximize therapeutic outcome and minimize cumulative toxicity. For example, cyclosporine can be thought of as a systemic parallel to halobetasol (ie, 'rabbit'), and acitretin viewed as the systemic counterpart of calcipotriene (ie, 'turtle'). Cyclospo-

Table 9-2: Sequential Therapy

Topical Sequential Therapy

Step 1

Calcipotriene (Dovonex®) + halobetasol (Ultravate®) twice daily (mixed immediately prior to application)

~2 weeks to 1 month

Systemic Sequential Therapy (Example 1)

Step 1	Step 2
Cyclosporine	Maintain cyclosporine and start acitretin. Optimize acitretin, then taper off cyclosporine.
~1 month	~3-6 months

Systemic Sequential Therapy (Example 2)

Step 1	Step 2
Cyclosporine	Maintain cyclosporine and start a biologic. When the biologic reaches optimal efficacy, taper off cyclosporine.
~1 month	3-9 months

PUVA=psoralen plus ultraviolet A; UVB=ultraviolet B

Step 2

Calcipotriene twice daily
on weekdays
Calcipotriene + halobetasol
twice daily on weekends
~1 month to indefinitely
for some patients

Step 3

Calcipotriene twice daily

Indefinitely or until
clearance*

Step 3A

Acitretin (Soriatane®)

Step 3B

Add UVB or PUVA.
Maintain on retinoids
with UVB (re-UVB) or
retinoids with PUVA
(re-PUVA).

Indefinitely or until
clearance*

Step 3

Maintain on a biologic.

Indefinitely or until
clearance*

*Depends on the natural history of psoriasis for the particular patient being treated.

rine is the agent of choice when rapid and significant clearing of disease is desired. Nephrotoxicity limits extended use of cyclosporine, and US Food and Drug Administration (FDA) guidelines mandate that uninterrupted treatment with this agent must be terminated after 1 year. Acitretin has less serious long-term toxicities and can be used safely for years. However, its onset of action is slow, and improvement is gradual. The side-effect profiles of cyclosporine and acitretin are dissimilar and metabolism is through differing mechanisms, so overlapping toxicity is minimal. Both can affect lipids, however, so the patient's fasting lipid profile needs to be monitored closely. Using the protocol below, clearance is rapidly achieved and safely maintained. The length of time the patient is on cyclosporine is decreased. Cyclosporine use and phototherapy are separated by a period during which the patient is on acitretin. This regimen might minimize the theoretical risk of skin cancer that is associated with using these two modalities together.

Step 1 consists of clearing the patient with cyclosporine at a maximum dermatologic dose of 5 mg/kg/day. A dose of 5 mg/kg/day is the maximum dosage recommended per international guidelines. The FDA recommends a maximum dosage of 4 mg/kg/day. Clearance or marked improvement of psoriasis might take approximately 1 month to accomplish, after which step 2 commences. The patient is maintained on cyclosporine for the next few months while therapy with acitretin is concomitantly initiated and optimized with respect to dosage. When the dosage of acitretin is maximized according to patient tolerance, the patient is gradually tapered off of cyclosporine. Step 3 consists of indefinite maintenance on acitretin alone. If this is not adequate to control the psoriasis, phototherapy can be added. Patients can be maintained on the retinoids with UVB (re-UVB) or retinoids with PUVA (re-PUVA) regimen for as long as there is adequate control of the psoriasis. If relapse occurs after this, enough time will have elapsed so that cyclosporine can be restarted and the sequence repeated.

These are the traditional examples of how sequential therapy can be used and regimens can be tailored to a patient's unique clinical situation. Other topicals, such as tazarotene (Avage®, Tazorac®), can be used in lieu of or in addition to calcipotriene. Systemic sequential therapy can be performed with any combination of an effective, rapid-acting agent combined with a drug that is safe to use long term for maintenance. For example, cyclosporine can be used in sequence with one of the newer biologic agents, such as etanercept or efalizumab.

Selected Readings

Koo JY: Sequential therapy of psoriasis. Introducing a new therapeutic paradigm for better clinical results. *J Am Acad Dermatol* 1999;41:S25-S28.

Koo J: How and why to employ sequential therapy for psoriasis. *Skin and Aging* 2000;(suppl):16-21.

Koo J: Systemic sequential therapy of psoriasis: a new paradigm for improved therapeutic results. *J Am Acad Dermatol* 1999;41 (3 pt 2):S25-S28.

Lebwohl MG: Combination, rotational, and sequential therapy. In: Weinstein GD, Gottlieb AB, eds: *Therapy of Moderate-to-Severe Psoriasis*, 2nd ed. New York, NY, Marcel Dekker, 2003, pp 179-196.

Lebwohl MG, Feldman SR, Koo JY, et al: *Psoriasis: Treatment options and patient management*. Portland, OR, National Psoriasis Foundation, 2002, pp 21-26.

CHAPTER 10

Advances in the Treatment of Psoriasis: The Biologic Agents

B iologic agents can be thought of as the strategic 'smart bombs' of the systemic immunomodulators. They are custom made and designed to interact with specific targets within the immune system, minimizing the collateral organ damage seen with the use of generalized immunomodulators, such as cyclosporine (Gengraf®, Neoral®, Sandimmune®) and methotrexate (Trexall™). The biologics are bioengineered proteins that bind to receptor sites on T cells or the cytokines they produce, blocking T-cell activation, killing T cells, blocking T-cell migration, or interfering with the action of cytokines and thereby inhibiting the inflammatory cascade.

Because the biologics are immunomodulators, there is concern about their potential to make patients more susceptible to infection or malignancy. The *Physician's Desk Reference*® and individual package inserts contain warnings about the possible increased risk of developing these adverse events. Indeed, rare cases of serious infection and malignancy have been reported with the use of each drug described in this chapter. However, not every biologic agent has shown convincing evidence of causing or increasing the risk of infection or malignancy.

A summary of biologic agents for psoriasis is presented in Table 10-1.

Alefacept

Alefacept (Amevive®) is a fusion protein combining a portion of human immunoglobulin (IgG) and the binding site of lymphocyte function-associated antigen-3 (LFA-3). It binds to CD2, the partner molecule of LFA-3 located on the surface of T cells. This drug also binds to the surface proteins of accessory cells, including natural killer cells and macrophages. Alefacept inhibits T-cell activation and proliferation and also induces T-cell apoptosis. Because it depletes a subset of CD4 T cells, the absolute CD4 count may decline and must be monitored during treatment.

Alefacept is administered via intramuscular (IM) injection. A dosing course consists of 12 weekly administrations of 15 mg IM. Absolute CD4 counts must be performed every other week during treatment, and the dose must be held if the CD4 count drops below 250 cells/mm^3. Patients can have repeated courses of alefacept, as long as their CD4 counts are within normal range and at least 12 weeks have elapsed between courses. Efficacy improves with each subsequent dosing course.

In an international, randomized, double-blind, placebo-controlled trial, Lebwohl et al evaluated the efficacy and tolerability of alefacept in 507 patients with chronic plaque psoriasis. Patients were given placebo, alefacept 10 mg, or alefacept 15 mg once a week for a total of 12 weeks. This study found that IM alefacept was well tolerated and effective, with 24% of the patients in the 15 mg group, 22% of patients in the 10 mg group, and 8% of the patients in the placebo group assessed as being clear or almost clear of psoriasis at 12-week follow-up. Mean Psoriasis Area and Severity Index (PASI) score reductions were 46% in the 15 mg group, 41% in the 10 mg group, and 25% in the placebo group at 6 weeks post-dosing.

In another double-blind, placebo-controlled, parallel-group study by Ellis et al, patients with chronic plaque psoriasis were given alefacept 0.025 mg/kg body weight,

Table 10-1: Summary of Biologic Agents Currently Approved by the FDA for Psoriasis

Drug	Dosing	Laboratory Tests, per FDA	Side Effects
Alefacept (Amevive®)	15 mg IM, office	CD4 counts every other week	Decrease in CD4$^+$ and CD8$^+$ T-lymphocyte counts
Efalizumab (Raptiva®)	Initial dose 0.7 mg/kg SC, followed by weekly dose of 1 mg/kg SC (maximum single dose not to exceed a total of 200 mg).	CBC and platelet counts recommended, but not required.	Flu-like symptoms Rebound upon discontinuation

CBC=complete blood count; IM=intramuscular; IV=intravenous; PPD=purified protein derivative; SC=subcutaneously

Current Indications	Efficacy Data
Psoriasis	During 24 wk of study, improvement in PASI ≥50% of baseline in 35%-57% (range) of patients, dose-dependent, and improvement in PASI ≥75% in 22%-33% (range) of patients, dose-dependent
Psoriasis	After 12 wk of treatment, improvement in PASI ≥50% of baseline in 52%-59% (range) of patients, and improvement in PASI ≥75% of baseline in 22%-39% (range) of patients

PASI=Psoriasis Area and Severity Index: a clinical assessment performed by physicians, which rates the overall severity of psoriasis based on erythema, plaque thickness, scaling, and affected body surface area (BSA).

(continued on next page)

Table 10-1: Summary of Biologic Agents Currently Approved by the FDA for Psoriasis *(continued)*

Drug	Dosing	Laboratory Tests, per FDA	Side Effects
Etanercept (Enbrel®)	50 mg SC twice weekly for the first 3 months. After first 3 months, 50 mg once weekly.	No tests are required by the FDA, but at individual clinician's discretion, PPD and other tests may be performed.	Injection site reactions
Infliximab (Remicade®)	Approved IV dose is 5 mg/kg body weight at 0, 2, 6 weeks, then every 8 weeks.	PPD pretreatment	Reactivation of TB Risk of infections Sepsis Opportunistic infections Rare cases of hepatosplenic T-cell lymphoma

IV=intravenous; PPD=purified protein derivative; PASI=Psoriasis Area and Severity Index; SC=subcutaneously; TB=tuberculosis

Current Indications	**Efficacy Data**
Psoriatic arthritis Rheumatoid arthritis Ankylosing spondylitis Plaque psoriasis Juvenile rheumatoid arthritis	PASI $\geq$75% in about 49% of patients in 12 weeks at 50 mg SC twice weekly.
Adult and pediatric Crohn's disease Plaque psoriasis Psoriatic arthritis Ankylosing spondylitis Ulcerative colitis	PASI $\geq$75% achieved by about 80% of patients in about 12 weeks at 5 mg/kg dosing.

0.075 mg/kg body weight, 0.150 mg/kg body weight, or placebo. This study used intravenous (IV) dosing, which was subsequently removed from the US market. The patients received one infusion/week for 12 weeks. Twelve weeks after treatment, 47%, 63%, and 42% of the three alefacept-treatment groups, respectively, had at least a 50% reduction in their baseline PASI scores. Of the patients who had received alefacept, 24% were clear or almost clear of psoriasis, compared with 5% of those patients who had received placebo.

While onset of action is slow, improvement with alefacept progresses over time, and patients typically continue to exhibit improvement even after the last dose of a course. Practitioners and patients should be realistic about how quickly they will see clinical benefit. Often, combination therapy with another relatively safe treatment, such as phototherapy, can be used to speed clearance initially, and then the response can be maintained over time with alefacept. A major benefit of alefacept is that it is a remittive therapy, and the median duration of response maintaining at least 50% improvement is 7 to 8 months among patients who achieve ≥75% improvement in PASI anytime during the 3-month treatment (injection) period or for 3 months after the treatment. With IM alefacept, 33% of patients achieve this level of improvement within the 6-month period described above. Alefacept is well tolerated, with no evidence of major organ toxicity or rebound after treatment has been completed. Of course, alefacept has only been studied for a few years, and long-term safety data is needed. Continued data collection spanning the course of 5 years or even decades is warranted and could be accomplished using a patient registry.

Because of its tolerability and favorable side-effect profile, alefacept may be well suited for long-term, intermittent use. It can also be a valuable agent for a patient who develops side effects from traditional systemic agents or who does not want to assume the potential risks associated with them. Alefacept is an especially useful option for a patient who has comorbidities for which medications such as methotrexate or cyclosporine are absolutely or relatively contraindicated.

Efalizumab

Efalizumab (Raptiva®) is a humanized monoclonal antibody directed against the T-cell surface molecule CD11a. The CD11a and CD18 proteins form lymphocyte function-associated antigen-1 (LFA-1), which plays a critical role in allowing lymphocytes to adhere to other cell types. Binding of efalizumab to CD11a blocks the interaction between LFA-1 and intracellular adhesion molecule-1 (ICAM-1), its partner molecule on the surface of antigen-presenting cells (APCs), vascular endothelial cells, and keratinocytes. Psoriasis-inducing T cells are thereby prevented from being activated in the lymph nodes or reactivated in the dermis and epidermis. ICAM-1's presence on endothelial cells also prevents T cells blocked by efalizumab from binding to the blood vessel wall and migrating into the skin.

Efalizumab is available as a subcutaneous preparation that patients self-inject once weekly. The recommended dose is a single 0.7 mg/kg subcutaneous conditioning dose followed by weekly subcutaneous doses of 1 mg/kg (maximum single dose not to exceed 200 mg). Dosing can be continuous with a good durability of response.

A trial conducted by Gordon et al found that 27% of patients who received efalizumab had a ≥75% improvement in PASI (ie, PASI 75) vs 4% of those in the placebo group at 12 weeks. This trial showed that, after 12 weeks of treatment, improvement in PASI ≥50% was found in 52% to 59% (range) of patients.

Another phase III trial conducted by Lebwohl et al found that at 12 weeks, 22% of patients who received efalizumab 1 mg/kg/week and 28% of those who received 2 mg/kg/week had a ≥75% or greater improvement in PASI, compared with 5% of those who received placebo. Statistically significant improvement was seen as early as

4 weeks after treatment began and PASI ≥75% improvement was maintained through week 24 in 77% to 78% of the patients who continued to receive efalizumab, compared with 20% of those who were switched to placebo. An improvement in PASI ≥50% was seen in 52% of the 1 mg/kg group and 57% of the 2 mg/kg group. After the drug was discontinued at week 24, one third of the patients maintained a ≥50% improvement in PASI during a 12-week follow-up period.

A third phase III trial, conducted by Menter et al, found that at week 12, 26.6% of the efalizumab-treated patients had a 75% improvement in PASI and 58.5% had a 50% improvement. At 24 weeks of continuous therapy, these percentages had increased to 43.8% in the 75% improvement group and 66.6% in the 50% improvement group. Recently, many cases of hand and foot psoriasis that responded well to efalizumab have been reported. A formal clinical trial on hand and foot psoriasis showed that efalizumab worked much better than the placebo. Exactly how efalizumab therapy for hand and foot psoriasis compares in efficacy with the traditional treatment options such as hand and foot PUVA phototherapy remains to be determined.

In clinical studies, efalizumab was well tolerated, with the most frequent side effects being transient, mild-to-moderate flu-like symptoms, including mild headache, fever, and chills. Acute adverse events occurred with the first dose, with the incidence decreasing with each subsequent dose. By the third dose, acute adverse events were not statistically different from placebo. Rare cases of thrombocytopenia, hemolytic anemia, and arthritis exacerbation have been reported with the use of this agent and therefore, the FDA recommends that patients have a CBC with platelet count once a month for the first 3 months and then at every 3-month interval. During clinical trials, after abrupt discontinuation of efalizumab, a small percentage of patients were noted to have recurrence of disease worse than baseline (rebound rate of 13.8% was noted in the clinical trial). This rebound can be minimized by formulating an appropriate transitional therapy strategy before discontinuation of the drug. In large, randomized, placebo-controlled clinical trials, efalizumab showed no evidence of cumulative or end-organ toxicity. Very rarely, some patients may experience sudden worsening of psoriasis while still being treated with efalizumab. If the worsening is only localized, topical therapy will usually suffice. If the worsening is generalized, then the best treatment option is cyclosporine.

Etanercept

Tumor necrosis factor-α (TNF-α) is a proinflammatory cytokine found in increased concentrations in the joints and skin. Endogenous skin cells and activated leukocytes secrete TNF-α, which binds to target receptors that are found on almost every cell of the body. TNF plays an active role in leukocyte recruitment, migration, and activation. Leukocytes activated by TNF secrete more cytokines, creating an inflammatory cascade.

Etanercept (Enbrel®) is a fusion protein consisting of two TNF receptors fused to the Fc portion of human immunoglobulin G (IgG) antibody. This construct creates an exogenous TNF receptor and prevents excess TNF from binding to cell-bound receptors. The end result is a reduction of active TNF and mitigation of diseases, such as rheumatoid arthritis and psoriasis, that are mediated by the effects of TNF. Etanercept has been used in approximately 500,000 patients with psoriatic arthritis over the past 15 years and is approved by the FDA for the treatment of psoriasis, psoriatic arthritis, ankylosing spondylitis, and juvenile and adult rheumatoid arthritis. A major benefit of this drug is that it halts the progression of bony destruction in psoriatic and rheumatoid arthritis while simultaneously treating the skin.

Although significant improvement of disease can be seen as early as 2 weeks after initiating therapy, the onset of action is gradual, with continued improvement over time. All efficacy measures are improved in a dose-dependent manner, including a mean improvement in skin score of up to 71% and quality of life (QOL) up to 74% (completely eliminating the effects of psoriasis on QOL in up to 25% of patients) after 24 weeks of therapy. Dosing can be continuous over years with a good durability of response. Alternatively, etanercept may be abruptly discontinued without risk of aggressive recurrence (rebound) of psoriasis. The most notable adverse event observed with therapy has been a transient, mild-to-moderate injection site reaction. Etanercept is FDA-approved for use in children with arthritis as young as 2 years. No laboratory monitoring is required by the FDA prior to initiation of, or during, etanercept therapy. However, physicians should use their own judgment in deciding what tests may be worthwhile for the patient on an individual basis. There have been rare reports of congestive heart failure exacerbation, bone marrow suppression, and conversion to positive antinuclear antibody during etanercept therapy, but a causal relationship with the drug has not been established because of the rarity of these cases. Extremely rare reports of demyelinating disease have also been associated with etanercept. Besides the absence of laboratory monitoring requirements and dosing flexibility, etanercept offers the added convenience of self-administration at home. For psoriatic and rheumatoid arthritis, patients inject 25 mg subcutaneously twice a week, at least 72 to 96 hours apart. This dose is also effective for psoriasis; however, if even greater efficacy or faster onset of action is desired, a dose of 50 mg twice a week has been extensively tested (in phase III clinical trials) and shown to have significantly enhanced efficacy in the skin with no increase in concern regarding adverse events.

Etanercept, for the treatment of psoriasis, has been approved for induction dosing of 50 mg subcutaneously twice a week for the first 3 months. After this 3-month induction phase, the dose of etanercept must be decreased to 50 mg once a week or 25 mg twice a week for maintenance regimen. However, some patients may deteriorate with regard to their psoriasis when the dose is decreased as specified by the FDA described above. Patients who are overweight or obese are at greater risk for deterioration in their psoriasis status as compared with patients who are not overweight. If deterioration occurs, the available options include enhancing efficacy with combination therapy, trying to go back to the higher dose even though this needs to be communicated to the patient as off-label treatment, or switch to another therapeutic option.

Infliximab

Infliximab (Remicade®) is a monoclonal antibody; this drug targets TNF and is administered intravenously. An initial infusion is given, followed by repeat administrations 2 and 6 weeks later. Patients can then be maintained with an infusion every several months. Infliximab is now indicated for the treatment of rheumatoid arthritis and Crohn's disease, ankylosing spondylitis, ulcerative colitis, psoriatic arthritis, and adults with chronic, severe plaque psoriasis who are not candidates for systemic therapy or when other systemic therapies are inappropriate. In September 2006, infliximab was approved for the treatment of psoriasis. Commonly reported side effects include nonspecific symptoms, such as headache and diarrhea. Screening for tuberculosis (TB) before starting therapy is particularly important because infliximab has been associated with rare incidents of reactivation of TB in patients with latent infection. A few cases of sepsis and opportunistic infections such as histoplasmosis have been reported with use of this agent, and it should be used cautiously in patients with congestive heart failure. A significant percentage of patients who take infliximab develop antibodies against the nonhuman portion of the drug. As a result, patients may need to take low doses of methotrexate concomitantly or be treated with infliximab every 2 months to suppress the development of these antibodies.

In studies of patients with moderate-to-severe psoriasis, infliximab has been shown to provide a rapid, durable response as well as a high level of sustained efficacy for at least 6 months. More research is needed to determine whether the initial level of efficacy can be sustained over extended periods with repeated exposure to infliximab, but current findings suggest that this agent may be an effective, remittive therapy for psoriasis. Consult the latest *Physician's Desk Reference*® for the full prescribing information on infiximab because several possible serious side effects ranging from rare cases of hepatotoxicity to hepatic cancers have been reported.

Selected Readings

Chaudhari U, Romano P, Mulcahy LD, et al: Efficacy and safety of infliximab monotherapy for plaque-type psoriasis: a randomized trial. *Lancet* 2001;357:1842-1847.

Ellis CN, Krueger GG, and the Alefacept Clinical Study Group: treatment of chronic plaque psoriasis by selective targeting of memory effector T lymphocytes. *N Engl J Med* 2001;345:248-255.

Gordon KB, Papp K, Hamilton T, et al: Efalizumab for patients with moderate to severe plaque psoriasis: a randomized controlled trial. *JAMA* 2003;290:3073-3080.

Gottlieb AB: Psoriasis. Immunopathology and immunomodulation. *Dermatol Clin* 2001;19:649-657.

Gottlieb AB, Hamilton T, Caro I, et al, and Efalizumab Study Group: Long-term continuous efalizumab therapy in patients with moderate to severe chronic plaque psoriasis: updated results from an ongoing trial. *J Am Acad Dermatol* 2006;54(4 suppl 1):S154-S163.

Gottlieb AB, Lowe NJ, Matheson RT, et al: Efficacy of etanercept in patients with psoriasis. Poster presented at American Academy of Dermatology, New Orleans, LA, Feb 22-27, 2002.

Intramuscular alefacept improves health-related quality of life in patients with chronic plaque psoriasis. *Dermatology* 2003;206:307-315.

Krueger GG: Clinical response to alefacept: results of a phase 3 study of intravenous administration of alefacept in patients with chronic plaque psoriasis. *J Eur Acad Dermatol Venereol* 2003;17: 17-24.

Krueger GG, Ellis CN: Alefacept therapy produces remission for patients with chronic plaque psoriasis. *Br J Dermatol* 2003;148: 784-788.

Krueger JG: The immunologic basis for the treatment of psoriasis with new biologic agents. *J Am Acad Dermatol* 2002;46:1-23.

Kupper TS: Immunologic targets in psoriasis. *N Engl J Med* 2003; 349:1987-1990.

LaDuca JR, Gaspari AA: Targeting tumor necrosis factor alpha. *Dermatol Clin* 2001;19:617-635.

Lebwohl M, Christophers E, Langley R, et al: An international, randomized, double-blind, placebo-controlled phase-3 trial of intramuscular alefacept in patients with chronic plaque psoriasis. *Arch Dermatol* 2003;139:719-727.

Lebwohl M, Tyring SK, Hamilton TK, et al: A novel targeted T-cell modulator, efalizumab, for plaque psoriasis. *N Engl J Med* 2003; 349:2004-2013.

Leonardi CL, Powers JL, Matheson RT, et al, and the Etanercept Psoriasis Study Group: Etanercept as monotherapy in patients with psoriasis. *N Engl J Med* 2003;349:2014-2022.

Mease PJ, Goeffe BS, Metz J, et al: Etanercept in the treatment of psoriatic arthritis and psoriasis: a randomized trial. *Lancet* 2000; 356:385-390.

Menter A, Gordon K, Carey W, et al: Efficacy and safety observed during 24 weeks of efalizumab therapy in patients with moderate to severe plaque psoriasis. *Arch Dermatol* 2005;141:31-38.

Papp K, Bissonnette R, Krueger JG, et al: The treatment of moderate to severe psoriasis with a new anti-CD11a monoclonal antibody. *J Am Acad Dermatol* 2001;45:665-674.

Pariser DM: Management of moderate to severe plaque psoriasis with biologic therapy. *Managed Care* 2003;4:36-44.

Singri P, West DP, Gordon KB: Biologic therapy for psoriasis: the new therapeutic frontier. *Arch Dermatol* 2002;138:657-663.

Tutrone WD, Kagen MH, Barbagallo J, et al: Biologic therapy for psoriasis: a brief history, II. *Cutis* 2001;68:367-372.

CHAPTER **11**

Nail Psoriasis

N ail changes are a common component of psoriasis and can be distressing for patients. For many patients, this is the only manifestation of their disease, making nail examinations and recognition of disease characteristics important aspects of clinical visits. Nail changes observed in psoriasis include oil spots, pitting, onycholysis, and subungual hyperkeratosis. Occasionally, patients will lose the entire nail (Figure 11-1, see color insert). Oil spots are semitransparent yellow or brown discolorations of the nail plate that were named because it looks like oil has seeped under the edge of the nail. Pitting is a deformity in which tiny, irregularly sized, shallow, round indentations are randomly distributed on the surface of the nail plate. Salmon spots are salmon-pink areas representing psoriatic involvement of the nail bed. Lifting of the nail plate, or onycholysis, is common, and refers to the separation between the nail plate and nail bed manifested by a whitish extension from the distal or lateral edge of the nail toward the cuticles. It is lined by an erythematous border marking the proximal edge. Onycholysis is often seen in conjunction with subungual hyperkeratosis.

Hyperkeratosis is also associated with fungal nail infections, which should be ruled out with cultures. One clinical difference is in the texture of the hyperkeratotic material. Hyperkeratosis of fungal infections is usually 'cheesier' and easily scraped off, while psoriatic hyperkeratosis is drier and more adherent.

Treatment of nail psoriasis is largely unsatisfying and counseling for these patients needs to be directed at setting appropriate expectations. Most treatments have either a high failure rate or unacceptable side effects. Nevertheless, some patients prefer to make an effort at amelioration and some do achieve success. Patient counseling should include a discussion that nail disease originates with an inflamed matrix, so any treatment that is successful will undoubtedly be slow because of the rate of nail growth. Patients should understand that the existing nail first must grow out before changes can be seen, which may take up to 1 year.

First-line agents for treating nail psoriasis include the topical therapies described in Chapter 5: calcipotriene (Dovonex®), and topical steroids, tazarotene (Avage®, Tazorac®), or anthralin (Drithocreme®, Psoriatec™); however, anthralin can stain the nail brown and topical steroids may induce atrophy of the surrounding skin. It is best to use combination regimens when treating nails, and many of these agents can even be applied simultaneously, as explained in Chapter 9. Much of the patient's treatment needs to occur overnight because of daily handwashing and inherent use of the hands. Patients can use either latex or cotton gloves to occlude their fingertips at night.

Nail matrix steroid injections can also provide some relief, although pain during injection and the risk of skin atrophy usually outweigh the benefits. Finally, systemic treatments such as methotrexate (Trexall™), or the newer biologics such as entanercept (Enbrel®), are helpful in treating nail involvement as well as skin and joint disease. Patients are rarely initiated on these treatments for nail involvement alone, but it could be done depending on the severity of disease, and the disfigurement, disability, and distress it causes the patient.

Selected Reading

Lowe NJ, Moy RL: Therapy of nail psoriasis. In: Lowe NJ, ed: *Practical Psoriasis Therapy*, 2nd ed. St. Louis, MO, Mosby-Year Book, 1993, pp 233-237.

CHAPTER **12**

Psoriatic Arthritis

P soriatic arthritis is more common than previously believed. Current surveys estimate that up to 20% of patients with psoriasis also suffer from joint disease. Among patients with moderate-to-severe psoriasis, up to 50% can present with significant arthralgias or formally diagnosed psoriatic arthritis. Although neither primary care physicians nor dermatologists are certified in rheumatology, recognizing symptoms and the presence of arthritis is within their capability. Often these providers serve as patients' only access to appropriate referral and joint care.

One critical difference between psoriasis and psoriatic arthritis is that psoriatic arthritis can lead to progressive and often irreversible bone and joint destruction, while psoriasis does not generate such permanent sequelae. To prevent this destructive process, it is critical for patients with early signs and symptoms of psoriatic arthritis to be identified and treated promptly, preferably with a safe agent known to alleviate symptoms and prevent progression of irreversible joint destruction (disease-modifying antirheumatic drugs [DMARDs], see below). Ask patients about morning stiffness, 'gelling' after rest, joint pain, joint swelling, fluctuations of these symptoms that correspond with changes in their skin, and family history of psoriatic arthritis. Constitutional symptoms are unusual in psoriatic arthritis. Patients should be examined for joint swelling, tenderness, reduced range of motion, as well as nail involvement, which often correlates with distal interphalangeal (DIP) involvement.

Table 12-1: Five Classifications of Psoriatic Arthritis

Type I   Asymmetric oligoarthritis
- Accounts for 70% of psoriatic arthritis
- Typically involves 2-3 small joints of fingers and toes
- Leads to 'sausage digits'
- Can involve bigger joints asymmetrically

Type II   Symmetric polyarthritis
- Clinically indistinguishable from RA
- Associated with low rheumatoid factor titers and elevated ESR
- Female preponderance

Type III   Classic psoriatic arthritis
- Involves DIP joints
- Associated with severe nail involvement
- Male preponderance

Type IV   Deforming polyarthritis
- Severe erosive disease
- Leads to arthritis multilans or 'pencil-in-cup' deformities, telescoping digits, and 'sausage digits'
- Involves DIP joints

Type V   Spondylitis/Sacroiliitis
- Involves sacroiliac and axial joints
- Male preponderance

DIP=distal interphalangeal; ESR=erythrocyte sedimentation rate; RA=rheumatoid arthritis

Psoriatic arthritis is a seronegative, inflammatory joint disease that can affect one or more joints, with a predilection for feet and hands, particularly the DIP joints (Figure 12-1, see color insert). Most patients present with skin disease first, but some present with simultaneous onset, and even fewer with joint disease that precedes skin disease. The latter diagnosis is a retrospective one, but patients complaining of joint pain should nevertheless be thoroughly examined for any sign of skin involvement, particularly in classic areas such as the umbilicus, scalp, gluteal cleft, elbows, knees, and nails to confirm the diagnosis.

There are five classifications of psoriatic arthritis (Table 12-1). The details of each are not as important as being able to recognize symptoms, which may indicate the presence of this disease and warrant a rheumatology referral. This is particularly important for primary care physicians and dermatologists who have the opportunity of seeing patients early in their disease process and prevent irreversible bony changes. Appropriate disease identification also allows for the selection of treatment that may be helpful for both skin and joints simultaneously.

Etanercept (Enbrel®) and infliximab (Remicade®), are FDA approved for the treatment of psoriatic arthritis, and are good choices for the treatment of both skin and joints. These agents are examples of a class of drugs called DMARDs, which are known to prevent or minimize the progressive bony destruction characteristic of psoriatic arthritis. Adalimumab (Humira®), which is currently FDA indicated only for psoriatic arthritis and not psoriasis, also has similar efficacy in preventing or minimizing the progressive bony destruction characteristic of psoriatic arthritis. Even though dermatologists and primary care physicians are not experts in rheumatology, it is perfectly acceptable to choose such systemic treatments rather than choosing a treatment that addresses only the skin (ie, topical medications, phototherapy). If possible, arthritis treatments that can complicate the management of psoriasis, such as systemic steroids, should be avoided. These are helpful tips in managing patients with psoriatic arthritis, but are not a replacement for individual management by a rheumatologist.

Selected Readings

Andrews BS, Lowe NJ: Therapy of psoriatic arthritis. In: Lowe NJ, ed: *Practical Psoriasis Therapy*, 2nd ed. St. Louis, MO, Mosby-Year Book, 1993, pp 239-256.

Gladman DD: Psoriatic arthritis. In: Weinstein GD, Gottlieb AB, eds: *Therapy of Moderate-to-Severe Psoriasis*, 2nd ed. New York, NY, Marcel Dekker, 2003, pp 219-237.

CHAPTER 13

Psoriasis in Pregnancy

Patients with psoriasis who become pregnant often experience significant improvement in their disease. One proposed etiology of this phenomenon is the bolus of natural hormones produced during pregnancy. This has also been used to explain the postpartum recurrence or rebound that women experience when their hormone levels suddenly plummet. However, women who experience continuation of their disease, or even exacerbation, during pregnancy require treatment.

For mild psoriasis, many patients prefer to use only nonmedicated emollients during pregnancy to reduce the risk of systemic absorption and fetal exposure to drugs, even those that are considered to be safe. An algorithm for patients requiring treatment is shown in Table 13-1.

For moderate-to-severe psoriasis, either ultraviolet B (UVB) phototherapy or bath-psoralen plus ultraviolet A (PUVA) (see Chapter 6) is acceptable, safe, effective treatment for psoriasis during pregnancy. UVB is usually suggested first because it is a simpler, less time-consuming treatment and does not involve the use of any chemical agents. Bath-PUVA is often reserved for more severe psoriasis because of the extensive time commitment required and low exposure to psoralen. Oral psoralens have not been shown to increase congenital malformations, although they may be associated with low birth weight. Although there is no convincing evidence that psoralen causes birth defects, the use of oral PUVA therapy is not recommended if pregnancy is an issue.

Table 13-1: Treatment Algorithm for Pregnant Patients	
First Line:	Topical medications (calcipotriene [Dovonex®] and topical steroids are Category C)
Second Line:	UVB phototherapy
Third Line:	Bath-PUVA
Fourth Line:	Goeckerman day care
Fifth Line:	Cyclosporine or biologics

PUVA=psoralen plus ultraviolet A; UVB=ultraviolet B

Goeckerman day care is an excellent option for its safety and efficacy, but is less attractive to many patients because of the inherent time constraints.

Cyclosporine (Gengraf®, Neoral®, Sandimmune®) can be used if necessary. Data collected from the national pregnancy registry of transplant patients who took the drug throughout their pregnancies shows that the drug is not teratogenic. Low birth weight and premature births were the only consistent findings in this group of patients. Nursing mothers should not use cyclosporine since it is secreted in breast milk.

Finally, several of the newer biologic agents such as alefacept (Amevive®) and etanercept (Enbrel®) are pregnancy Category B.

Physicians need to be aware not only of appropriate treatment options during pregnancy, but also which drugs are contraindicated (Table 13-2). Oral retinoids, such as isotretinoin (Accutane®) and acitretin (Soriatane®), as well as the topical retinoid tazarotene (Avage®, Tazorac®) are Category X and absolutely contraindicated during pregnancy, in women of childbearing age who do not use

Table 13-2: Treatments That Are Contraindicated During Pregnancy

Oral retinoids:	Category X	Acitretin (Soriatane®)
		Isotretinoin (Accutane®)
Topical retinoids:	Category X	Tazarotene (Avage®, Tazorac®)
Methotrexate:	Category X	Trexall™

The same guidelines should be used for women who do not use adequate birth control or who are planning to become pregnant.

---

adequate birth control, or in those who plan to become pregnant within 3 years of use in the case of acitretin. The half-life of acitretin, the only oral retinoid now approved for the treatment of psoriasis, is approximately 50 to 100 hours. However, ingestion of alcohol during therapy promotes transesterification of acitretin to etretinate, which has a half-life of 120 days, and can be detected in the serum up to 2 years after discontinuation of treatment.

The topical retinoid approved for psoriasis is tazarotene. Although it is Category C in other countries, it remains Category X in the United States. This is because of possible systemic absorption of the drug and fear of teratogenicity as seen with the use of oral retinoids. As with oral retinoids, women should have a pregnancy test before starting treatment and use adequate birth control throughout treatment.

Methotrexate (Trexall™) is known and used as an abortifacient. It can be teratogenic at low doses and is strictly contraindicated during pregnancy. Women should not take this drug during pregnancy and should not become pregnant for at least 1 month after discontinuation. Many physicians use a more conservative recommendation of 2 to 3 months. Because of reports of sperm abnormalities, the same recommendation is made for men regarding fathering a baby while they are taking methotrexate and for several months afterward.

CHAPTER 14

For the Nonspecialist: When to Refer

Treating psoriasis with topical agents in patients whose disease involves >10% of total body surface area is usually not feasible. To estimate involvement, use the size of the patient's palm plus their fingers and thumb, which is approximately 1% of their total body surface area. Generally, nondermatologists have little expertise with phototherapy or other systemic agents for the treatment of psoriasis. Therefore, while it is still important to prescribe topical medications, it is equally important to recognize that patients with >10% body surface area involvement should be referred to a dermatologist for more definitive treatments such as phototherapy, systemic therapy, or Goeckerman therapy (see Chapter 8).

In some cases, even when involvement is <10%, psoriasis may be resistant to maximal topical regimens, or the patient may find his or her disease particularly distressing. In these cases, referral is appropriate for more creative therapeutic combinations or more sophisticated modalities. Systemic therapy may be appropriate in mild cases in which a patient's quality of life (QOL) is severely disturbed because of the disease. Even small, recalcitrant lesions in sensitive areas, such as the scalp, genitalia, gluteal cleft, or hands, can be physically or emotionally disabling.

If the patient has significant problems with arthralgias or arthritis, referral to either a dermatologist, rheumatologist, or both is appropriate. Certain systemic treatments can be beneficial for skin and joint disease. Some of the newer bio-logic agents such as etanercept (Enbrel®) may be the safest available treatments for this disease combination.

Index

A

Abelcet® 52
Accutane® 54, 91, 92
acitretin (Soriatane®) 51, 54, 56, 62, 64-68, 91, 92
Aclovate® 24
acne 26, 33
acyclovir (Zovirax®) 52
Adalat® 50
Adalat® CC 50
adrenal suppression 21, 28, 30, 64, 65
Aggrenox® 49
Alavert® 12
alclometasone 25
alcohol 5, 20, 47, 92
alefacept (Amevive®) 64, 71, 72, 76, 91
Alkeran® 53
alopecia 57
AmBisome® 52
amcinonide 23
Amevive® 64, 71, 72, 91
aminoglycosides 49
ammonium lactate 32
Amphotec® 52
amphotericin B (Abelcet®, AmBisome®, Amphotec®) 52
anemia 56

angiotensin-converting enzyme (ACE) inhibitors 6
anthralin (Drithocreme®, Micanol®, Psoriatec™) 18, 35, 36, 60, 85
antibiotics 45
antidepressants 45
antifungals 51
antihistamines 12
antihypertensives 50
antimalarials 6
antipsychotics 45
Aquaphor® 60
Aralen® 6
arthralgias 86, 94
arthritis 7, 46, 78, 86, 94
asthma 9, 46
atopic dermatitis 5, 8, 9, 12
atrophy 13
Avage® 18, 60, 69, 85, 91, 92

B

β-blockers 5, 6
bacterial infections 9, 13
Bactrim™ 48, 49, 52
barbiturates 48, 49
betamethasone 23, 25, 27
biologic agents 42, 59, 63, 66, 67, 69, 70, 72, 74, 85, 91, 95

bipolar disorder 6
birth control 55, 92
birth defects 90
body surface area (BSA) 15, 42, 73
bone marrow suppression 47, 48, 56, 57, 63, 64
breast milk 91
broadband UVB 44
bromocriptine (Parlodel®) 53
burning 30, 34, 43-45

C

Calan® 51, 53
calcipotriene (Dovonex®) 11, 15, 18, 19, 27-31, 32, 34, 35, 38, 39, 60, 64, 65, 67
cancer 7
candidiasis 9
Capex® 24
carbamazepine (Tegretol®) 6
Cardene® 53
cardiac failure 13
Cardizem® 51, 53
Cataflam® 53
Category X 47, 55
cephalothin 49
chills 13
chloroquine (Aralen®) 6
cimetidine (Tagamet®) 53
cirrhosis 53
Claritin® 12
clobetasol 23, 27-29, 34
Clobex® 22, 28
coal tar 18, 36, 37, 59, 60
colchicine 49
cold weather 5
complete blood count (CBC) 47, 50, 54, 56, 57
congenital malformations 90

contact dermatitis 9
contraception 35
Cordran® 21, 22, 24
Cormax® 22
corticosteroids 6, 13, 46, 53, 64
Coumadin® 53
Cutar Emulsion® 36
Cutivate® 22, 24
Cyclocort® 22
cyclosporine (Gengraf®, Neoral®, Sandimmune®) 29, 48, 50-52, 56, 62-65, 68, 70, 91
cytokines 6, 48

D

danazol 53
Daraprim® 49
decreased night vision 53
Depakote® 6
depression 7, 54
dermatitis 5, 9-12, 26
dermatologists 14, 25, 29, 32, 34, 42, 44, 48, 50, 54, 86, 88, 94
Dermatop® 24
desonide (DesOwen®) 25
DesOwen® 24
desoximetasone 23
diabetes 7
diclofenac (Cataflam®) 53
diffuse idiopathic skeletal hyperostosis (DISH) syndrome 54
diflorasone (Psorcon® E™) 23, 27
Diflucan® 52
digoxin (Lanoxin®) 51
Dilantin® 48, 49

diltiazem (Cardizem®)
51, 53
Diprolene® 22, 27
Diprosone® 22
dipyridamole (Aggrenox®,
Persantine®) 49
disease-modifying
antirheumatic drugs
(DMARDs) 86
diuretics 45, 51
divalproex (Depakote®) 6
dizziness 44
Dovonex® 11, 15, 18, 29,
60, 64, 85
doxycycline (Vibramycin®)
52
Drithocreme® 85
Droxia® 55, 56, 64
dust 9
DynaCirc CR® 51
Dyrenium® 49

E

eczema 8, 10-12, 27
dyshidrotic eczema 11
eczematoid psoriasis 10, 11
efalizumab (Raptiva®) 64,
69, 72, 77, 78
Elidel® 18
Elocon® 22, 27
Enbrel® 16, 64, 74, 79, 85,
88, 91, 95
Epitol® 6
Ery-Tab® 52
erythema 8, 11, 12, 26, 30,
38, 39, 51, 73
Erythrocin® 52
erythromycin (Ery-Tab®,
Erythrocin®) 52

Eskalith® 6
etanercept (Enbrel®) 16,
29, 69, 74, 79, 80, 85, 88,
91, 95
ethanol 49, 55
etretinate 92

F

Fansidar® 49
fever 13
fibrosis 53
Florone® 22
fluconazole (Diflucan®) 52
fluocinonide (Lidex®) 23,
25, 27, 31
flurandrenolide tape
(Cordran® tape) 21, 25
fluticasone 23, 25
folliculitis 26, 38
fungal infections 9, 84
Fungizone® 52
furosemide (Lasix®) 53

G

gastrointestinal disturbance
57
gemfibrozil (Lopid®) 6
Gengraf® 29, 48, 56, 62, 63,
70, 91
gentamicin (Garamycin®)
52
gingival hyperplasia 51
gluteal pinking 8
Goeckerman (inpatient)
therapy 59, 60, 91, 94
Goeckerman day-care
centers 38
granulomas 53

H

H$_2$-blockers 51
hair loss 53
halcinonide 23
halobetasol (Ultravate®)
    23, 27, 64-66
Halog® 22
hand and foot psoriasis
    14, 42, 52, 58, 78
headaches 44, 47, 51, 53
heart disease 7
heart failure 7, 14
heliotherapy 45
hepatotoxicity 47, 57, 64
histamine 12
human immunodeficiency
    virus (HIV) 49
Hydrea® 55, 56, 64
hydrocortisone 23-25
hydroxychloroquine
    (Plaquenil®) 6
hydroxyurea (Hydrea®)
    55, 56, 63, 64
hypercalcemia 31
hyperkeratosis 11, 38, 84
hyperlipidemia 51, 57
hyperostosis 54, 57
hyperpigmentation 57
hypertension 7, 48, 50, 57
hypertrichosis 26, 51, 57
hyperventilation 39
hypoglycemia 40
hypopigmentation 26

I

induration 12, 38
infliximab (Remicade®)
    74, 81
inpatient therapy 59
interferons 6

interleukin-2 (IL-2) 48
irritation 13, 30, 32, 34, 36,
    38
Isoptin® SR 51, 53
isotretinoin (Accutane®) 54,
    91, 92
isradipine (DynaCirc CR®)
    51
itching 20, 34, 44
itraconazole (Sporanox®) 52

J

joint pain 88
joints 88

K

Kenalog® 22
Keralyt® gel 38, 39
keratinocytes 77
keratolytic 38
ketoconazole (Nizoral®) 52

L

lactic acid 18, 32, 40, 59, 60
Lanoxin® 51
Lasix® 53
lesions 6, 8, 10-14, 30, 46
leukocytosis 56
Lidex® 22, 27
light exposure 43
light therapy 47, 59
lipid profile 50, 54, 57, 68
liquor carbonis detergens
    (LCD) 36, 37, 39, 60
lithium (Eskalith®, Lithobid®)
    5, 6
Lithobid® 6
liver biopsy 47, 48, 57
liver function tests 47
liver toxicity 48

Locoid® 24
loop diuretics 45
Lopid® 6
loratadine (Alavert®, Claritin®) 12
lovastatin (Mevacor®) 51
low birth weight 90, 91
lung disease 7
lymphoma 47, 49

M

maceration 13
macrocytosis 56
malaise 47
malignancy 49, 70
melanoma 44
melphalan (Alkeran®) 53
methotrexate (Trexall™) 29, 46-49, 51, 55, 56, 64, 70, 92
metoclopramide (Reglan®) 53
Mevacor® 51
micaceous scales 8, 10
mometasone 23, 27
mood disorders 54
myalgias 53
mycosis fungoides (MF) 9-11

N

nails 9, 84-87
    nail bed 9
    nail infections 84
    nail plate 84
    nail psoriasis 14, 46, 84, 85, 87
    pits 9, 84
nausea 39, 44, 47, 51
Neoral® 29, 48, 56, 62, 63, 70, 91

nephrotoxicity 48, 50, 57, 68
Neutrogena® T/Gel® Shampoo Extra Strength 39
nicardipine (Cardene®) 53
nifedipine (Adalat®, Procardia®) 50
Nizoral® 52
nonsteroidal anti-inflammatory drugs (NSAIDs) 6, 48, 49
norfloxacin (Noroxin®) 52
Noroxin® 52
Nutraderm® 37

O

onycholysis 9, 84
oral contraceptives 51, 52, 55

P

pain 20, 85
paresthesias 51, 57
Parlodel® 53
peeling 30
penicillin 49
Persantine® 49
petrolatum 37
pets 9
pharmacist 35
pharyngitis 13
phenylbutazone 49
Phenytek® 48, 49
phenytoin (Dilantin®, Phenytek®) 48, 49
photosensitivity 38, 43, 44, 47
phototherapy 32, 36, 42, 43, 45, 47, 51, 55, 60, 62, 63, 68, 94
pimecrolimus (Elidel®) 18

pityriasis rosea 9
pityriasis rubra pilaris (PRP) 9, 10
plaque-type psoriasis 12, 13, 14, 28, 33, 46, 71
Plaquenil® 6
plaques 8, 10-12, 20, 28, 33, 35
pneumonitis 47
pollen 9
prednicarbate 25
prednisone 51
premature births 91
primary care physician 48, 86, 88
Probalan® 48, 49
probenecid (Benemid®, Probalan®) 48, 49
Procardia® 50
Procardia® XL 51
Protopic® 18
pruritus 12
pseudotumor cerebri 55
psoralen 90
psoralen plus ultraviolet A (PUVA) 11, 43, 44, 50, 52, 54, 60, 63, 66, 67, 90, 91
   bath-PUVA 43, 90, 91
   oral-PUVA 43
   paint-PUVA 43
Psorcon® E™ 22, 27
psoriasiform eczema 10, 11
psoriasis 5-9, 11-14, 18-21, 25, 27-30, 33, 36, 38, 44, 46, 48, 49, 51, 59, 67, 82, 84, 86, 90, 92, 94
   erythrodermic 12, 13, 46, 48
   guttate 13
   hand and foot 14, 42, 52, 58, 78

psoriasis *(continued)*
   in pregnancy 90-93
   nail 14, 46, 84, 85, 87
   plaque-type 12-14, 28, 33, 46, 71
   prevalence 5
   pustular 13, 14, 46, 52
   scalp 14, 20
   von Zumbusch type 14
Psoriasis Area and Severity Index (PASI) 32, 59, 73, 76, 77
Psoriatec™ 18, 85
psoriatic arthritis 16, 46, 75, 79, 80, 86-88
psoriatic lesions 8, 10, 46
psoriatic plaques 24, 36, 39
psoriatic skin 6
pulse therapy 27, 65
pustular psoriasis 13, 14, 52
pyrimethamine (Daraprim®, Fansidar®) 49

Q

quality of life 80, 94
quinacrine 6

R

ranitidine (Zantac®) 53
Raptiva® 64, 72, 77
rash 10
re-PUVA 52, 54, 67
re-UVB 52, 54, 67
rebound 46
Reglan® 53
Remicade® 74, 81
renal dysfunction 48
renal failure 13, 14
renal toxicity 56
Retin-A® 33

retinoids 33, 35, 49, 51, 52, 54, 62, 63, 91, 92
rheumatoid arthritis 75, 79-81, 87
rhinitis 9
rigors 13
rosacea 26

S

salicylates 49
salicylic acid 18, 32, 37, 38, 59, 60
salicylism 39
salmon spots 9, 84
Sandimmune® 29, 48, 56, 62, 63, 70, 91
scales 8, 10, 11, 38
scaling 12, 73
scalp psoriasis 14, 20
seborrhea 8, 10
seborrheic dermatitis 8, 9, 27
sepsis 14
Septra® 48, 49, 52
skin and joint disease 95
skin antigen testing 9
skin atrophy 21, 24, 28, 32, 34, 64, 65, 85
skin biopsy 11
skin cancer 44, 50, 54, 63, 68
Soriatane® 51, 56, 60, 62, 91, 92
sperm abnormalities 93
Sporanox® 52
steroids 11, 18, 20-22, 24, 26, 27, 29-34, 39, 64, 65, 85, 89
stinging 34
stress 5
stretch marks 21
striae 21, 26, 30

suicide 54
sulfonamides 48, 49
sulfonylureas 49
sunlight 45
Synalar® 22, 24

T

'tapioca' vesicles 11
T-cell lymphoma 9, 10
tachyphylaxis 27
Taclonex® 32
tacrolimus (Protopic®) 18, 19
Tagamet® 53
tanning beds 45
tar preparations 18, 36-38, 59, 60
tazarotene (Avage®, Tazorac®) 18, 32, 33, 35, 39, 60, 69, 85, 91, 92
Tazorac® 18, 60, 69, 85, 91, 92
T cells 6, 48
Tegretol® 6
telangiectasias 26
Temovate® 22, 27
teratogenicity 57, 92
tetracycline 49, 55
thiazide diuretics 53
thrombocytopenia 56, 78
tinea 9
tinnitus 39
Tobi® 52
tobramycin (Tobi®) 52
toenails 85
topical agents 18, 19, 26, 33, 35, 36, 42, 94
Topicort® 22
tretinoin (Retin-A®) 33
Trexall™ 29, 46, 56, 64, 70, 85, 92

triamcinolone 23, 27
triamterene (Dyrenium®)
49
Tridesilon® 24
trimethoprim/
sulfamethoxazole
(TMP/SMX) (Bactrim™,
Septra®) 49, 52
tumor necrosis factor-α
(TNF-α) 79

U

Ultravate® 22, 27, 64, 66
ultraviolet A (UVA) phototherapy 32, 42, 44, 63
ultraviolet B (UVB) phototherapy 11, 32, 35, 42, 43,
52, 54, 59, 60, 63, 66, 67,
90, 91
  broadband UVB 44
  narrow-band UVB
  42-44

ultraviolet light 42
US Food and Drug Admin-
istration (FDA) 19, 25, 28,
33, 38, 46, 50, 55, 68, 79

V

Valisone® 22, 24
verapamil (Calan®, Isoptin®)
51, 53
Vibramycin® 52
viral infections 9
vitamin A 33
vitamin D 29
vomiting 47

W

warfarin (Coumadin®) 53
Westcort® 22, 24

Z

Zantac® 53
Zovirax® 52

Contemporary Diagnosis and Management of Psoriasis®

Retail $22.50

Ordering Information

Prices (in U.S. dollars)

1 book:	$22.50 each
2-9 books:	$20.25 each
10-99 books:	$18.00 each
> 99 books:	Call 800-860-9544*

How to Order:

1. by telephone: 800-860-9544*
2. by fax: 215-860-9558
3. by Internet: www.HHCbooks.com
4. by mail: Handbooks in Health Care Co.
       3 Terry Drive, Suite 201
       Newtown, PA 18940

Shipping/Handling

**Books will be shipped via Priority Mail
or UPS Ground unless otherwise requested.**

1-3 books:	$6.00
4-9 books:	$8.00
10-14 books:	$11.00
15-24 books:	$13.00
> 24 books:	Plus shipping

International orders: Please inquire

*Please call between 9 AM and 5 PM EST Monday through Friday, 800-860-9544.

Pennsylvania residents must add 6% sales tax.

Prices good through September 30, 2008